Lecture Notes on Traun

Lecture Notes on Trauma

Edited by John Templeton FRCS
Consultant Orthopaedic Surgeon

and R.I. Wilson MBE, FRCS
Former Professor of Orthopaedic Surgery

Division of Orthopaedic Surgery
Musgrave Park Hospital
Belfast

Blackwell Scientific Publications

OXFORD LONDON

EDINBURGH BOSTON MELBOURNE

© 1983 by
Blackwell Scientific Publications
Editorial offices:
Osney Mead, Oxford OX2 OEL
8 John Street, London WCIN 2ES
9 Forrest Road, Edinburgh EH1 2QH
52 Beacon Street, Boston
  Massachusetts 02108, USA
99 Barry Street, Carlton
  Victoria 3053, Australia

First published 1983

Set by Colset (Pte) Ltd, Singapore
Printed and bound in Great Britain
by Billing and Sons Ltd, Worcester

DISTRIBUTORS

USA
  Blackwell Mosby Book Distributors
  11830 Westline Industrial Drive
  St Louis, Missouri 63141

Canada
  Blackwell Mosby Book Distributors
  120 Melford Drive, Scarborough
  Ontario, M1B 2X4

Australia
  Blackwell Scientific Book Distributors
  31 Advantage Road, Highett
  Victoria 3190

British Library
Cataloguing in Publication Data

Templeton, J.
  Lecture notes on trauma.
  1. Wounds and injuries
  I. Title   II. Wilson, R.I.
  617'.21   RD93

  ISBN 0-632-01043-6

Contents

Contributors, vii

Preface, ix

**Section 1   Emergency management of
a seriously injured patient**

Introduction, 3
1   Resuscitation, 5
2   Diagnosing the full extent of the injuries and management, 6
    Head injuries, 8
    Neck injuries, 17
    Chest injuries, 19
    Abdominal injuries, 25
    Pelvic injuries, 32
    Thoraco-lumbar spinal injuries, 41
    Limb injuries, 42
3   Drug Treatment, 47
4   Mobilisation of staff, 53
5   Making a good record, 54
6   Monitoring the patient's condition, 55

Section 2   Injury to specific parts

7   The eye, eyelids and orbit, 61
8   Ear, nose and throat, 69
9   The shoulder, 73
10   The elbow, 76
11   The wrist, 79
12   The hand, 83
13   The hip, 85
14   The knee, 93
15   The ankle, 95
16   The foot, 97
17   Shafts of long bone, 100

Section 3

18   Vascular injuries, 107
19   Fractures in children, 132
20   Open fractures, 136
21   Burns, 138
22   Amputations and orthotics, 142

Index, 146

Contributors

Ian V. Adair FRCS, Consultant Orthopaedic Surgeon

Desmond B. Archer FRCS, Professor of Ophthalmology

David St C. Baird FRCS, Consultant Orthopaedic Surgeon

Aires A.B. Barros D'Sa MD FRCS, Consultant Vascular Surgeon

Dermot P. Byrnes FRCS, Senior Lecturer/Consultant Neurosurgeon

James W. Calderwood FRCS, Consultant Orthopaedic Surgeon

D.L. Coppel FFARCS, Consultant Anaesthetist

John M. Gorman FDSRCS, Consultant Oral Surgeon

John A. Halliday BSc FRCS, Consultant Orthopaedic Surgeon

W.V. James FRCS, Consultant Orthopaedic Surgeon

Alan G. Kerr FRCS, Consultant ENT Surgeon

John H. Lowry FRCS, Consultant Orthopaedic Surgeon

Roy Millar FRCS, Consultant Plastic Surgeon

R.A.B. Mollan FRCS, Professor of Orthopaedic Surgery

Alastair L. Macafee MD FRCS, Consultant Orthopaedic Surgeon

Norman W. McLeod FRCS, Consultant Orthopaedic Surgeon

James R. Nixon MChOrth FRCS, Consultant Orthopaedic Surgeon

Paul H. Osterberg FRCS, Consultant Orthopaedic Surgeon

J. Piggot FRCS, Consultant Orthopaedic Surgeon

J.B. Pyper FRCS, Consultant Orthopaedic Surgeon

G.F.W. Price FRCS, Consultant Orthopaedic Surgeon

C.F.J. Russell FRCS, Consultant Surgeon

W.H. Rutherford OBE FRCS, Consultant in Accident and Emergency

H.M. Stevenson FRCS, Consultant Thoracic Surgeon

Trevor C. Taylor FRCS, Consultant Orthopaedic Surgeon

Maureen J. Turtle MB BCh, Consultant in Accident and Emergency

All contributors practise at one or more of the following: Altnagelvin Hospital, Londonderry; Belfast City Hospital, Lisburn Road, Belfast BT9 7AB; Musgrave Park Hospital, Balmoral, Belfast BT9 7JB; Royal Victoria Hospital, Grosvenor Road, Belfast BT12 6BA, Northern Ireland.

Preface

To the layman TRAUMA often means psychological insult. In medicine it usually refers to non-psychological injury. It is therefore a very broad subject involving all surgical specialities to a lesser or greater extent. These notes are written at a clinical student level and therefore deal with principles rather than detailed management.

Several decades ago R.J.W. Withers, who founded the orthopaedic service in Northern Ireland, produced a synopsis of 'Fractures'. This synopsis gave invaluable assistance and confidence to generations of medical students. It has been completely revised and its base broadened to include Trauma to all parts of the body to become *Lecture Notes on Trauma*. Section 1 deals with the management of the seriously and usually multiply injured patient. Section 2 deals with injuries to more specific and isolated parts of the body. Section 3 covers a miscellaneous group of important problems related to trauma.

Acknowledgements

Lecture Notes on Trauma could not have been produced without the many contributions from our Consultant colleagues. We would also like to thank Mrs Marie Loughran for her tireless secretarial assistance.

Section 1
Emergency management of a seriously injured patient

Introduction

Sometimes a junior doctor finds himself a member in a team looking after a severely injured patient. He is then allocated a specific task and if any difficulties arise he can turn immediately to a senior colleague. It is not uncommon, however, for a junior doctor to find that he is the only person present when the patient arrives. His main difficulty in this situation is that he has several different kinds of responsibilities. These cannot be taken up and discharged one after another. All need to be kept in mind simultaneously and progress is made gradually on several different fronts. It is dangerous to become too deeply engrossed in any one aspect to the exclusion of others.

In the first sixty seconds there are three main tasks:
1 To transfer the patient to an accident trolley without aggravating any injuries. This is fairly easy when the patient is on a lifting sheet. Be ready to use wooden poles to increase the rigidity of the sheet while lifting. If there is no lifting sheet hand lift the patient with three people at the side and one at the head of the patient. Lift the patient straight upwards and stand still, holding up the patient. The first trolley is pulled away and a second inserted. The patient is lowered on to it. *Never* put two trolleys together or attempt to half lift, half push the patient sideways.
2 Remove *all* clothing. Taking off clothes is quicker than cutting but with unstable neck or spine injuries or other very painful situations, cutting is necessary.
3 Get a detailed description of the accident from the ambulance man or any available witness.

With the patient on the accident trolley there are now six main tasks:
1 Resuscitation.
2 Diagnosing the full extent of the injuries and management.
3 Drug treatment.
4 Mobilising medical staff
   (a) To help in the immediate resuscitation.
   (b) To take over the further care of the patient.
5 Making a good record.
6 Monitoring the patient's condition.

1 Resuscitation

Put your cheek and ear close to the patient's nose and mouth, at the same time looking along the chest wall. Make sure you can feel and hear air moving in and out. Is the chest wall moving? Is it moving in the right way, rising on inspiration and falling on expiration? Does the patient look at all blue? Remember that an anaemic patient can be severely hypoxic without being blue. In bad facial injuries, it may be best to allow the patient to sit and lean forwards.

For unconscious patients the usual options, after sucking blood and vomit away, are an oral airway, a nasopharyngeal airway and an intratracheal tube. Where the patient is deeply unconscious he will allow the passage of an intratracheal tube immediately. Otherwise, the passage of an intratracheal tube will usually require a general anaesthetic. Occasionally only a tracheostomy will secure a satisfactory airway. One or two 14 guage catheters passed through the crycothyroid membrane will give temporary relief and allow the tracheostomy to be done in a more cool and controlled manner.

Any obvious external haemorrhage should be controlled by a firm pressure dressing. It is wise to insert an intravenous cannula in all seriously injured patients. As the injuries are diagnosed, the blood loss is estimated and blood ordered. Infusion can be started with Hartman's solution or Haemaccel, of which up to two litres may be given before starting blood. Always use the largest possible cannula, usually No. 14. Try arm veins first. If they are collapsed, immerse the arm in warm water. In cases of difficulty, the subclavian vein is very useful. For cut downs, use the cubital fossa. For rapid infusion set up two or three lines.

2 Diagnosing the full extent of the injuries and management

This is a matter of a careful and systematic examination of the whole patient, head to toe, front, sides and back.

Re-checking the history

At this point, the more information that is available on exactly how the accident happened the better. If this aspect of the history has not yet been elucidated, it is well to see whether the patient, any other patient in the same accident, an ambulance man or any other available witness can describe in detail the mechanism of injury.

Cleaning up

Immediately after the injury the extent of the injuries may be obscured by the presence of blood or dirt. It is often worth cleaning the skin quite thoroughly. Unsuspected wounds and other injuries may become evident.

The patient with localised injuries

Not infrequently it is very evident roughly where the injury lies. If a girder falls and traps a man, crushing his right thigh and producing a compound fracture of the femur, this will be immediately evident. Gunshot wounds will often present with one or two small circular wounds. A boy stabbed in the chest with a knife may present with two or three linear wounds over his lung or heart. In such cases it is often possible to confirm within a few seconds that the remainder of the body is uninjured. The patient confirms that he has no pain, no tenderness and no loss of function elsewhere. All attention can then be given to the vicinity of the injury. Often one should look for both primary injury and for the presence or absence of a secondary injury (e.g. is there a fracture and is there any secondary damage to nerves or vessels?).

The patient suspected of multiple injuries

In some accidents the whole body has been exposed to external forces,

6

and it is not possible immediately to know which parts of the body are or are not injured (the most usual example is a car occupant in a road traffic accident). The history may still help. The stationary car struck from the back by a speeding vehicle is the typical mechanism for a whiplash injury of the neck. A belted front seat passenger in a head-on crash is a possible candidate for a ruptured duodenum. The unbelted patient, especially if he is thrown through the windscreen or out the door is in danger of receiving a whole series of contacts with the car, the road, and other objects on or near the road. In this type of injury it is essential to approach the examination in a methodical manner, trying to think of and then either confirm or exclude a whole series of injuries.

The examination will have established already the patency of the airway, the adequacy of respiratory movements and signs of normal blood volume or hypovolaemia, as these are looked for in the early stages of resuscitation.

X-ray examination

Where the patient's condition is stable

Full examination of every suspected area may be carried out. It is justifiable to move the patient towards the X-ray room where the best facilities for radiography are available.

Where the patient's condition is unstable

Ideally the X-ray room will be adjacent to the resuscitation room and one examination room designed as an extension of it. Where this is not so, it may be necessary to keep the patient in the resuscitation room and use a portable X-ray machine. In unconscious patients with possible trunk damage, X-rays of chest, abdomen and pelvis should be taken. Where spinal injury is expected, spine X-rays are immediately necessary. For the neck remember to visualise C7. With suspect injuries to urethra and bladder, ascending urethrogram and cystogram should be considered. If the chest X-rays show a broad mediastinum, repeat pictures and even an angiogram of the aortic arch may be indicated.

HEAD INJURIES

The prospect of recovery from head injury is dependent on three major factors:
1 Severity of the injury.
2 Age of the patient.
3 Quality of medical care.
Only the third of these can be influenced.

Given that physical brain injury cannot be undone in the reconstructive sense, management is essentially the provision of the best possible environment for recovery, should recovery be possible. What is this best possible environment? Essentially this consists of being sure that the brain is being supplied by oxygenated red cells, especially that part which has been injured. This supply must be continuous and secure. Anything which interferes with it, be it a pneumothorax, hypotension or an extradural haematoma, must be prevented or diagnosed and treated.

The first priority therefore is the provision of an efficient airway. The airway can be compromised not just by foreign bodies, such as food or vomit, but simply by the lack of protective reflexes which the unconscious patient may exhibit. Any head injury patient who is not awake or apparently close to it should probably have an endotracheal tube inserted. This in most cases is relatively easy and a technique which all Casualty officers should be familiar with. At least one intravenous line must be erected. This is necessary for drugs and infusions should they be required. However, unless the patient needs a volume replacement immediately — and primary closed head injured patients seldom do — do not overinfuse. It is best simply to keep the intravenous line open until fluid requirements have been estimated. If the patient is hypotensive or in shock then this must be countered immediately no matter what the head injury problem is. Once airway and circulation have been stabilised then a rapid neurological assessment can be done. This must be simple, relevant and automatic. Estimate and record the level of consciousness *in words*; what the patient can do — answer questions? follow commands? respond purposefully to pain? Do not express level of consciousness in ambiguous terms, such as drowsy, unconscious, in coma, and do not say what the patient *cannot* do. Accompany this by a record of pupil size, reaction and laterality — i.e. movement symmetry about the midline and vital signs. In the deeply unconscious a word about brain stem reflexes such as breathing, corneal reflex and caloric response is valuable.

It can be seen from the foregoing that the first steps are not specifically neurological at all but simply the standard procedure in resuscitation from any cause. Try now to obtain some history from relatives or ambulance personnel. At this stage laboratory and X-ray studies can be considered. Arterial blood gasses are the most valuable immediately. These can be accompanied by haemoglobin estimation, blood glucose, electrolytes and grouping with a crossmatch for an arbitrary four units of blood. Serum osmolality and toxicology screen can also be helpful.

Turning to X-ray, the first should not be a skull series. Lateral cervical spine to include C7 followed by chest X-ray are initially the most important. Both are best done, if in any doubt as to the patient's stability, by portable equipment in the Resuscitation Room. Look for cervical spinal injury and pneumothorax.

Following this skull X-rays can be done, usually an AP, a lateral and a Towne view to look for a fracture, foreign body, intracranial air or evidence of a calcified pineal gland (shift of the last from the midline may help in the diagnosis of an intracranial haematoma). Further X-rays can be taken as required (e.g. a depressed fracture).

In some head injury cases, particularly if the level of consciousness is below brisk bilateral purposeful response to pain, steroids are usually given intravenously. This prescription is almost universal but its effect is unproven and there is increasing opinion which suggests that rather than be helpful they may actually be detrimental to the patient in terms of wound healing and infection. Mannitol should not be given nor should a lumbar puncture be performed without direct discussion with a neurosurgeon.

Bleeding from the nose and mouth can be controlled by packing and is seldom a severe problem. Brain tissue from the nose or mouth should be noted and covered but is not to be regarded as a hopeless sign. It simply means that a frontal or temporal lobe and dura have been lacerated. The use of prophylactic antibiotics is controversial especially in open wounds including cerebrospinal fluid leak. A good case can be made against them.

Deterioration of level of consciousness is an emergency. It does not necessarily mean an expanding intracranial clot; other conditions such as hypoxia, an epileptic fit, sedative medication, even hypovolaemia may be the cause. If the deterioration is not immediately attributed to one of these causes, then an extradural or subdural expanding haematoma must be suspected and acted upon. The usual diagnostic steps are a computerised tomography (CT scan) or angiography. In the absence of these facilities very occasionally diagnostic burr holes (close to a fracture, for instance) may be done on the side of a dilating pupil. This drastic step is seldom necessary and more time spent on airway and circulation will save more lives in the long run.

In summary the initial steps in the management of head injuries are theoretically simple, being the provision of adequate airway and circulation, the recording of neurological status and the surveillance for deterioration.

Facial injuries

The examination for injury to the facial bones and jaws is undertaken *after* the establishment of a clear airway and the control of haemorrhage.

Simple measures such as sucking out blood clot from the mouth and nostrils, and pulling forward the tongue and broken jaw fragments will help to clear the airway. Avulsed teeth and fragments of dentures should be looked and felt for, and removed. The upper jaw may be displaced backwards, and it can be pulled forwards away from the tongue by finger traction around the back of the hard palate. Nasopharyngeal tubes in both nostrils are often more valuable than an oral airway which may be poorly tolerated and easily displaced.

The position of the patient is all important, and the patient lying on his back may asphyxiate because the jaw fragments and tongue fall back to close the airway. The World War I dictum of 'if you are looking up to heaven you will soon be there' is still to be remembered. The ambulant patient is usually most comfortable if seated with the head bent well forwards so that gravity will help the tongue and jaws to fall forwards, and blood and saliva to drain out of the mouth. The seriously injured patient should lie on one side with a leg flexed or, if on a stretcher, in the prone position with the forehead supported by a belt and bandages stretched from handle to handle. If simple measures are not working then an oral endotracheal tube should be passed after which a decision on a tracheostomy can be made. Oedema can become very marked in gunshot wounds and this should be anticipated by the early passing of a tube.

The facial bones, jaws and dentition are readily accessible for examination. While facial oedema can mask injury, a great deal can be learnt from inspection and palpation of the bony margins and contours and of the inside of the mouth, provided that the examiner has a working knowledge of surgical anatomy and of the usual fracture patterns. While a full radiographic examination should be done it may be impractical to request a large number of views of a seriously injured patient. For such patients a few general radiographs of the cranium, facial bones and neck should be taken as a first step. For mandibular injuries the radiographs needed are P.A. and lateral oblique views of each side. If an orthopantomograph is available, and if the patient is ambulant, an overall view of the mandible and the lower part of the upper jaw can be obtained. This view is useful as one side of the mandible can be compared with the other, and dislocation of the condyle head easily recognized.

Surgical anatomy

For descriptive purposes the face can be conveniently divided into thirds. The upper third lies above the orbits, the middle third is from the supra-orbital margins above to the occlusal plane of the maxillary teeth below, and the lower third is from the occlusal plane to the lower border of the mandible.

Middle third

The middle third of the facial skeleton has over 20 constituent bones related to the orbital and nasal cavities, and the mouth. The *MAXILLAE* are the largest of these bones and are situated in a central position forming the upper jaw and palate below, enclosing the maxillary antra, making the walls of the nasal (pyriform) aperture, and being the main part of the orbital floors above. They articulate laterally with the *ZYGOMATIC (MALAR)* bones which contribute to orbital floors and the inferolateral part of the orbital rims, and which articulate with the frontal bones above and the temporal bones behind.

The structure of the middle third is well designed to withstand the occlusal load on the teeth and to distribute it over a wide area of the cranium. It is not so well adapted to take force from its front or laterally, and such force can cause considerable damage. Looked at from the side the facial bones and cranium meet along an inclined plane of approximately 45 degrees. Because of this when the facial bones as a whole are broken off the cranial base they may be displaced as much downwards as in a backwards direction. Clinically, this gives the effect of lengthening as well as dishing of the face.

Fractures involving the orbit may cause a change in position of the globe of the eye by altering the position of the attachments of the suspensory ligament. Further, if there has been comminution of the orbital floor, or of the ethmoids, herniation of periorbital tissue may occur, and this will give enophthalmos. Where such damage occurs without orbital rim fracture the injury is known as a 'blow-out fracture'.

The infra-orbital nerve lies first in a groove and then in a canal in the orbital floor and passes on to the cheek through the infra-orbital foramen. This foramen lies close to the junction of the maxilla and zygoma.

Mandible

The mandible is the largest and strongest of the facial bones. It is made up of a rounded horseshoe-shaped body which meets at the back on either side a flat ascending ramus. It articulates with the maxillae through the dentition and with the base of the skull through the temporomandibular joints. The articular condyles are attached to the ascending rami by slim condylar necks. The teeth are supported by alveolar bone set on top of the main body of the mandible. The nerve supply, the inferior dental nerve, enters the medial side of the ramus at the mandibular foramen and ends in the incisive and mental nerves, the latter nerve going out through the mental foramen to supply the lower lip and chin on each side.

Fracture patterns and clinical features

Middle third fractures

The most minor middle third fracture is an alveolar fracture where one or more teeth with supporting bone is broken off the maxilla, and the most major will be a craniofacial disjunction where the facial bones as a whole are sheared off the cranial base. The best working classification of these fractures was given by Le Fort in 1901 after experimental work. He divided the fractures into three basic types, but the clinician has to remember that he will meet many differing combinations of these fracture patterns.

Le Fort I. This is a low transverse fracture involving principally the antral walls and nasal septum in which the upper teeth, alveolus, and palate are separated from their base. The upper jaw may be mobile or displaced and impacted with derangement of the bite (dysocclusion). When the upper teeth are percussed a peculiar 'cracked teacup' sound is heard and this always presents in upper jaw fractures. Because the fracture line is below the infra-orbital foramina there is no facial anaesthesia nor are there black eyes, major nasal fracture, or widespread facial oedema.

Le Fort II. This is a pyramidal block fracture of the central part of the middle third. The pyramid has the teeth and palate at its base and the interorbital-ethmoidal region as its apex. The nasal bridge and infra-orbital rims will be fractured, as will be the maxillary walls in the region of the maxillary zygomatic suture and infra-orbital foramina.

Le Fort III. This is a high transverse fracture giving a craniofacial disjunction. The main fracture line will run across from one zygomatico-maxillary suture to the other affecting the orbits, nasal bones and ethmoids in its path. While this transverse line may be the only major fracture, the Le Fort III is more commonly seen in combination with other patterns. For example both the molars may be separated off, and there may be Le Fort I and II fractures also present with a palatal split. There is usually oedema giving a 'football face' which may mask the dishing and lengthening of the face which the displacement gives in Le Fort II and III fractures. The back teeth may meet abnormally causing the front teeth to lie apart with the upper teeth in an obviously inward displaced position.

In a Le Fort II fracture the central part of the middle third may be mobile as a whole. This should be tested for bimanually, moving the upper jaw and feeling for transmitted movement at the nasal bridge. The whole face in a Le Fort III may be loosened and can be moved from side to side as well as in a forwards direction. Bruising about the eyes with sub-conjunctival haemorrhages in them are a usual feature due to orbital rim fracture. Such fractures may be felt as steps along the lower and lateral parts of the orbital margin. In severe fractures there may be displacement of one or both eyes. The eyelids may be very swollen and it is often necessary to hold them apart to test for pupil level and vision. Diplopia and oculo-paresis may be found.

Damage to the cribriform plate of the ethmoid with an associated dural tear will give rise to CSF rhinorrhoea. There is then the danger of meningitis and of air escaping into the anterior cranial fossa. Permanent damage to the olfactory nerves may occur with this fracture.

Fracture of the zygoma

1 Zygomatic arch fracture can occur where the orbital margin is not involved, and where the arch may be pushed down on top of the coronoid process of the mandible.
2 Fractures of the zygoma also appear with the fracture sites usually close to the articulations with the frontal, temporal and maxillary bones.

In these fractures there may be considerable limitation of opening of the mouth due to bone fragments pressing on the coronoid process. Inward displacement is common and the contour of the cheek and arch should be looked at and felt, and comparison made with the cheek on the opposite side. A convenient way is to look at the patient from above and behind, and to use the arch of the forehead as a base line to compare the prominences of each cheek. The orbital rims should be carefully palpated and steps will often be found approximately midway along both the inferior and lateral margins. Due to fracture at, or close to, the infra-orbital foramen, there is often numbness of the cheek and lateral side of the nose, with also associated numbness of the upper teeth.

Eye injury such as was described for mid-third fractures may be present, and subconjunctival haemorrhage and bruising are usual features.

Mandibular fractures

Fracture of the alveolar bone with one or more teeth is the commonest injury, and in this the teeth with the supporting bone are sheared off the body of the mandible. Because the mandible is curved there are frequently two or even three fractures from one impact. For example, a blow on the side of the chin may cause indirect fractures at the angle or condylar neck on the opposite side, as well as a direct fracture. A fall or blow at the front of the chin often fractures the symphysis and both condylar necks. Compression of the jaw from side to side may fracture both angles and the symphysis. The junction of body to ramus is a place of relative weakness and this is often accentuated by the presence of a buried wisdom tooth. The condylar necks are also weak and are common fracture sites. If this were not so, there would be more danger of the condylar head being driven into the middle cranial fossa.

In contrast to middle third injuries, where force and its direction are all important in causing displacement, in the mandible it is the fracture sites and resultant muscle pull on the fragments which are the main factors giving displacement. The elevator muscles work on the rami, and the depressors on the body of the mandible. This means in bilateral angle fractures that there would be upwards and forwards rotation of the rami, with a depression of the body. It is this fracture which carries special risk to the airway if the patient is on his back, because the tongue and body of the mandible fall back to close the pharynx. At the fracture site there will be swelling and bruising. Depending on the displacement there may be noticeable deformity or asymmetry of the mandible. Jaw movement is usually restricted and may be abnormal when movement is attempted. Palpation from one condyle to the other along the lower border will detect fracture sites because of tenderness, or step defects, or alteration in contour such as the inward displacement of the angle.

Facial wounds may mean that the fracture is compound externally and, if the teeth are involved, the fracture will be compound into the mouth. The fact that a fracture is compound intra-orally may go unrecognized and lead to infection. Where the body of the mandible has been fractured to give damage to the inferior dental canal and its contents, there will be paraesthesia or anaesthesia in the distribution of the mental nerve. This will be noticed as altered or absent sensation in the lower lip and chin on the injured side.

Treatment

In general terms the treatment of facial and jaw fractures is the same as for all fractures, being directed towards proper reduction, adequate fixation, prevention of infection, and restoration of function. So that function can be restored the teeth have to be brought back into occlusion, and if this is not done there will be mal-union, dysocclusion and poor function.

Middle third fractures

1 External fixation. Maxillary complex fractures are stabilised by craniomaxillary or craniomandibular fixation. The teeth are immobilised in occlusion (termed intermaxillary fixation or IMF) and fixation is done with extension rods from dental splints or from mandibular pins held to either supra-orbital pins or a cranial headcap.

2 Intermaxillary fixation (IMF). Suitable for some Le Fort I and II fractures with little mobility or displacement.

3 Internal fixation by means of wires from dental splints below to fixation points above in the frontal or zygomatic bones.

4 Open reduction, where often in addition to other fixation methods, the various fracture sites are exposed and directly wired.

Zygomatic fractures

1 External operations through the Gillies temporal approach (using a lever under the arch) or via the face (placing a hook under the zygoma).

2 Intra-oral operation passing a suitable lever under the zygoma.

3 Stabilisation by means of wiring the fracture sites, external pins, antral packing or silastic wedges internally, or by passing a Kirschner wire from the sound side.

Mandibular fractures

1 Interdental and eyelet wiring. Eyelet wires are placed on both sets of teeth and the the teeth are wired up in the position of occlusion to give IMF.

2 Arch bars and silver cap splints may be used for IMF.

3 Where there are no teeth the dentures can be modified, wired onto the jaws and then fixed together.

4 Open reduction and bone wiring which is usually done with IMF.

5 Bone plating is useful where there are no teeth, or where because of other injury IMF is contraindicated.

6 External pins used with connecting rods to maintain alignment.

Treatment of soft tissue injuries

Where facial wounds are also present these should be dealt with *after* reduction of the fractures. The surgeon must always work from the inside outwards, replacing the tissues where they normally belong. If there has been tissue loss, as is likely in blast injury, the defect should be accepted at the time, and reconstruction carried out to a definite plan later.

NECK INJURIES

Injury to the neck may involve the major vessels, nerves, trachea and cervical spine. Vascular injuries are dealt with in Section III. Injury to the trachea will cause massive surgical emphysema. With neck wounds, remember the possibility of the wound tract running downwards to the thorax and occasionally upwards to the head.

Cervical spine

In general terms the understanding, diagnosis and treatment of spinal injuries is dependent on the stability of the vertebral segments and the presence or absence of neurological damage. If the injury has been such as to cause instability then the careful handling of the patient during transfer, examination and nursing procedures is necessary in order to prevent injury to the contents of the spinal canal or further damage if this has already occurred. The ability to influence the recovery of damaged spinal segments at a fundamental level is extremely limited. It can perhaps be modified by returning the spinal canal to maximum diameter and alignment quickly after injury and reducing cord oedema pharmacologically.

Injuries to the cervical spine are mainly caused by hyperflexion forces resulting in dislocations of the facetal joints or fracture-dislocations. These are very unstable injuries and the patient must be treated with caution. Vertical compression fractures or bursting fractures of the vertebral bodies, may occur when a force is transmitted down the spine from a blow to a fall onto the vertex. These injuries are essentially stable but may result in neurological damage if disc material or bony fragments are displaced into the spinal canal. Hyperextension injuries usually occur in older age groups and are often found in the presence of cervical spondylosis. The neurological pattern is variable with more disability in the upper limbs than the lower.

Many patients suffering a high cord lesion develop paralysis of the respiratory muscles and appear to be in respiratory distress. As a result many are nursed in the 'coma' position with the head rotated to one side thus increasing pressure on the spinal cord. The correct position is to lay the patient supine with the head extended and the chin supported. This position ensures the airway and improves the spinal canal diameter. It is the start of treatment.

A careful history will often reveal the mechanism of injury and a complaint of neck pain should be seriously noted followed by palpation of the neck for mid-line tenderness. If an injury is suspected then it must be considered as unstable until proven otherwise. Neurological examination is essential and in these circumstances is best performed starting distally, examining movement and sensation in the feet and toes, then working proximally to examine the major muscle groups in the legs and finally the arms. Sensory loss should be carefully recorded (a body map is useful). Perineal and perianal sensory sparing is an important finding; in the meantime, temporary immobilisation can be achieved between sandbags.

Adequate X-ray examination is essential and is complicated by the fear of endangering the patient while manipulating the cassettes. This can be partially overcome by ensuring that an X-ray trolley is used in Casualty and that a responsible member of the emergency team is always present to steady the head and to exert manual traction if any movements are required. It must be remembered that the cervicothoracic junction is often difficult to visualise and yet must be adequately complete. The patient with an obvious clinical injury but apparent normal spinal alignment should have a film taken with the neck flexed to ensure spinal stability. In those with marked muscle spasm this may not be immediately possible and may require some days bed rest before sufficient relaxation is obtained. Ignoring this detail can result in late, progressive slipping of the vertebrae and chronic spinal cord pressure. The significant abnormalities on routine radiographs are the loss of alignment of the posterior aspect of the vertebral bodies and widening of the interspinous distances. These are pathognomonic of instability. Vertical compression force to the neck may cause burst injuries, which are stable but may cause neurological damage through bony fragments being squeezed posteriorly into the spinal canal. These fragments can be clearly seen on X-ray.

Before any further movement of the patient the neck must be adequately stabilised. This can best be achieved by the attachment of skull traction, preferably using skull calipers. All doctors working in emergency areas should be familiar with their application. Once attached the possibility of further damage to the spinal cord is considerably reduced.

In the patient with a neurological injury the care of the skin and bladder is important from the outset. Insensitive skin can develop pressure ulceration extremely rapidly and once established may take many months to heal, affecting the whole rehabilitation process adversely. Once skull calipers have been applied with traction, the patient can be log-rolled at regular intervals to relieve pressure from the back and buttocks. The heels should be padded. The paralysed bladder distends and overstretching delays the return of tone to the bladder muscle. If the patient is seen to be quadriplegic then a small self-retaining catheter should be inserted and open drainage permitted. Extreme antiseptic care should be taken in this procedure because infection once introduced into the paralysed bladder is rarely removed.

The dislocated neck should be reduced as soon as possible after injury, preferably within the first few hours. This is most quickly performed by manipulation under anaesthetic when the vertebral bodies and facetal joints are easily realigned. In some situations anaesthesia is contraindicated for other reasons and in this situation the addition of increasing weight to skull traction combined with sedation will usually be successful. The patient must be carefully monitored during this procedure while the weight is built up rapidly to 40–50 lbs. and frequent lateral X-rays are taken. Once reduction has been obtained, the weight may be reduced to a holding level of 5–7 lbs. In the patient with a neurological deficit, particularly if incomplete, consideration must be given to bone or soft tissue impingement at the cord even when alignment appears satisfactory. The patient can be rolled on to his face while the neck is kept extended by placing the forehead on a sand-bag and traction continued. A lumbar puncture needle is then inserted from the side to enter the subarachnoid space between C1 and C2. Myodil is then gently layered into the cerebrospinal fluid and it trickles down the posterior aspect of the vertebral bodies into the cervical lordosis. A portable X-ray machine at the bedside will be sufficient to visualise any defect in the Myodil column produced by an anterior obstruction. If this is present then emergency anterior decompression and cervical fusion is essential. In the patient with a complete neurological lesion or an unstable spine but no cord damage, then cervical fusion for stability may be performed electively.

CHEST INJURIES

Chest injuries are common and may be divided into:

1 *Closed Injuries* commonly follow road accidents. Usually part of a multiple injury pattern, with damage to chest wall or diaphragm and possible injury to thoracic viscera.

2 *Penetrating Injuries* are usually the result of gunshot wounds or knife wounds. Damage of varying severity to pulmonary or mediastinal structures may be caused.

Closed injuries

Such injuries are usually multiple, so that the driver of a car involved in an accident may have spectacular but relatively unimportant cuts on the face, a stove-in chest, and fracture of one or both legs. The pedestrian is more likely to be struck on the back or side of the chest, and children who are run over often suffer abdominal or pelvic injuries, but may get into severe respiratory difficulty from an associated rupture of the diaphragm.

The actual chest injury may vary from a simple fracture of one or more ribs, to multiple fractures leading to an unstable fragment of chest wall, with or without a fracture of the sternum. Damage to the lung or bronchi leads to leakage of air, producing either a pneumothroax or haemothorax, and surgical emphysema. Cardiac contusion may result in diminished output, though ECG changes are very variable. Rupture of the aorta, which may be delayed, may follow severe compression injuries, and is sometimes associated with a fracture of the thoracic spine.

Even after a simple fracture of one rib, there is a partial shutdown of the pulmonary circulation in the underlying lung. In severe cases, this leads to increasing loss of function of the whole lung, even though respiratory movements continue, and even though the lung may be essentially undamaged. Several other factors greatly aggravate the pulmonary state, such as reflex pulmonary vasoconstriction, consequent upon extra-thoracic injury, low blood volume and large transfusions of either crystalloid solution or blood. Pain leads to suppression of cough, and associated head injury may abolish the cough reflex altogether. Secretions accumulate in the bronchial tree, which may also contain blood, and vomited material may be aspirated. An unstable fragment of chest wall leads to paradoxical respiration, and the presence of a pneumothorax or haemothorax further interferes with ventilation.

Thus, there is a lethal triad of bleeding, drowning and suffocation. Significant bleeding into the chest may be overlooked, as even a substantial quantity of blood in the pleural cavity may appear insignificant on a chest X-ray and there may be massive loss of blood into the abdomen from visceral injury, or around long bone fractures. The patient is literally drowning in the secretions of his bronchial tree, and being suffocated by the extra pulmonary effects of an unstable chest wall, haemothorax and pneumothorax, particularly if the latter is associated with tension. These features are interdependent. Inadequate ventilation and attempts to remove secretions, requires an increase in the cardiac output, which a patient with blood loss cannot achieve. Likewise paradox, and above all pain, prevent the patient from coughing up these secretions. This cycle of events, if untreated, leads to cardiorespiratory failure and death.

Treatment

One's approach to treatment should be somewhat similar to that of head injuries, in that it is more important to try and assess the effect of injury, rather than its extent. The vital feature which must be monitored is adequacy of ventilation. In the case of a simple rib fracture in a young, fit individual, careful clinical and X-ray examination is essential to exclude pneumothorax. If there is a pneumothorax, then a large size intercostal tube should be inserted, preferably in the second intercostal space anteriorly in the mid-clavicular line. Any area of localised surgical emphysema always indicates some pulmonary damage. Pain relief in such a case may be obtained with local anaesthesia or oral analgesics, or controlled intravenous analgesia if the patient is to be admitted. If he is allowed to go home, he should always be seen the next day, but admission should be advised in the presence of any complications, however trivial, or if the patient is old or bronchitic. In more serious cases, however, more definitive measures are required.

First aid management

This depends to some extent upon the skill of personnel at the scene of the accident, and enquipment available. Essential measures are:
1   Clear airway.

2 Maintain adequate ventilation with mouth to mouth respiration or Ambu bag.

3 Occlude any open wound.

4 Control external bleeding.

5 Control paradox with a firm pad and bandage.

Providing that ventilation can be maintained satisfactorily, and that the patient's general condition is being assessed by a doctor, intravenous analgesia may be given at this stage, the dose and drug given, and time of administration recorded. An accident flying squad should therefore be trained and equipped to:

1 Pass an endotracheal tube.

2 Institute pharyngeal and tracheal suction.

3 Set up an intravenous infusion.

4 Administer intravenous analgesic drugs.

Initial hospital management

First aid measures should be continued. An endotracheal tube should be passed, and the tracheobronchial tree cleared by suction. Some sedation should be given, having regard to whether or not any drugs have been given at the scene of the accident, but such sedation should be short of full anaesthesia. This is important, as full examination for other injuries, especially abdominal, is impossible if the patient is anaesthetized. The patient should be transfused, and a clinical check made for blood or air in the pleural cavities. A chest drain or drains should be inserted as necessary, which should be connected to calibrated underwater seals, so that blood loss from the chest may be recorded, and an estimate made of the amount of air leakage from damaged lung or bronchi. An erect chest X-ray should now be taken, though this may precede the insertion of chest drains if the patient's condition permits. Other injuries may now be evaluated and attended to and an estimate made, including blood gas studies of the patient's ventilatory state, following the measures taken.

On the basis of these observations a decision must now be made as to whether the patient's ventilation should be controlled with relaxants and Intermittent Positive Pressure Respiration instituted. This will almost certainly be necessary where there is severe paradox and other major injuries such as head injuries are present, but it should not be undertaken routinely, as long-term ventilation has its own morbidity and mortality.

Indications for thoracotomy in closed chest trauma

1 Excessive leakage of air, either from drainage tube inserted to relieve pneumothorax, or manifest as mediastinal emphysema, generally due to tear of trachea or bronchus.

2 Excessive and continuing intrathoracic haemorrhage.

3 Where ruptured diaphragm is suspected.

Ruptured trachea and bronchus

Note the significance of surgical emphysema which is mainly mediastinal in type. The maximal effects are notable in the head and neck, where it may be very tense. There may or may not be associated pneumothoraces. Increasing mediastinal emphysema is due to a valvular type of tear of a major air passage, aggravated by retained secretions and attempts to cough. The passage of an endotracheal tube often relieves this valvular mechanism, if it is at tracheal level, but diagnostic bronchoscopy is essential. Major tracheobronchial injuries are rare, but certain features are of diagnostic interest. The great majority of such patients are under forty years of age, 50 per cent of them have no other injuries, and chest wall injury occurs in only 33 per cent, this being usually fracture of some or all of the first three ribs. Initial treatment is as for other serious chest injuries, but open thoracotomy with expert anaesthesia will be required to close the tear.

Excessive and continued intrathoracic haemorrhage

This may be due to a ruptured aorta, which is leaking into the pleural cavity. Frank haemorrhage, however, may be delayed, as the tear is temporarily contained by the adventitia leading to a false aneurysm. In such cases a triad of symptoms may be present, falling Hb, hypertension, and a large pulse pressure. On chest X-ray there is widening of the upper mediastinum and serial films may show that such widening is increasing. While mediastinal widening of itself is not diagnostic, since it may be due to a large substernal haematoma in any severe chest injury, the possibility of aortic rupture should nonethless be suspected, and appropriate investigations carried out. Aortography is the only certain method of diagnosing this condition, but this should not be undertaken until the operating theatre is prepared for surgery. Aortic rupture characteristically occurs just distal to the origin of the left subclavian artery, and where it is proven, urgent surgical repair is indicated.

Ruptured diaphragm

Rupture of the diaphragm is one of the most urgent of surgical emergencies, which may be unsuspected for the simple reason that it is seldom associated with injury to the chest, but gives rise to a serious intrathoracic problem. In cases of blunt trauma, it accompanies sudden or crushing injuries to the abdomen or pelvis, and the onset of increasing dyspnoea in association with such injuries should always raise the possibility of diaphragmatic rupture. The sequence of events is that abdominal viscera, especially the stomach, may herniate through the diaphragmatic defect. Obstruction of both the cardia and outlet of the stomach occur, with increasing gastric distension, collapse of the lung, and displacement of the mediastinum to the opposite side. These effects may be more rapid where the tear is comparatively small; where a complete tear occurs, distension of the viscera does not take place, and the diagnosis may be made at a much later date. It is the left diaphragm which is almost always involved, and in addition to increasing dyspnoea, the patient may complain of nausea, and often retching or vomiting. There may be left shoulder tip pain.

On examination the apex beat is displaced to the right, the left chest is tympanitic and bowel sounds may be audible in the chest. There is often considerable intrathoracic and intra-abdominal bleeding from the diaphragm and possible associated damage to the spleen, and there is guarding of the left upper abdomen. The diagnosis is confirmed by an erect chest X-ray. This is an absolute indication for surgery, but the initial treatment is important.

1 Pass gastric tube. This may help to prevent gastric distension but in some cases it may not be possible to pass a tube into the stomach because of angulation at the cardia.

2 If distension of the stomach is extreme and a tube cannot be passed, then the stomach should be aspirated through the chest wall as an emergency measure prior to thoracotomy.

3 The patient should not be ventilated with a mask, as this increases gastric distension. If ventilatory assistance is required, an endotracheal tube should always be passed.

Penetrating injuries

In such injuries, success depends more upon speed of admission to hospital, and emergency care on arrival, than upon any other factor. Blood loss may be severe and a large intravenous cannula should be inserted, in order that the blood volume may be restored and maintained. A CVP line should also be inserted, since excessive transfusion can be extremely harmful in this situation. The same general principles apply as in the early management of closed chest injuries, and a chest drain is inserted into one or both pleural cavities where obvious penetration by a missile has occurred, or where there is any clinical evidence of blood or air in the pleural cavity. In gunshot wounds, an estimate is made of the probable track of the missile or missiles, and careful clinical examination is carried out, especially of the abdomen. Low velocity missiles are often retained, and X-ray films of chest and abdomen should be taken, and should accompany the patient to the operating theatre. While some knife wounds of the chest may be trivial, where cardiac injury is suspected, urgent thoracotomy is required, in view of the possibility of massive bleeding, with or without cardiac tamponade.

Indications for surgery in penetrating injuries

Absolute indications for surgery in penetrating chest injuries are:
1 Significant or continued haemorrhage.
2 A dangerous predicted track.
3 Associated intra-abdominal injury.
While some penetrating injuries may be managed with simple chest drainage under constant observation, it is evident that, on the basis of these criteria, surgical exploration of the chest, and often of the abdomen also, may be required.

ABDOMINAL INJURIES

Closed injuries

Injuries may be masked especially in the unconscious patient. On first assessment the most important information is the history of the accident which may be obtained from the patient, from friends and relations, from ambulance crew or from the police. Useful information includes blood loss, the change in the patient's condition, the type of accident and the forces of injury, whether any medicines have been given since the injury and the normal state of health of the patient. Any injury to the abdominal wall or its surrounding bony cage may be accompanied by serious injury to the abdominal viscera. Conversely the viscera may be damaged without any external evidence of injury to the abdominal wall. The abdominal viscera may be injured directly or indirectly. Different modes of trauma may result in a variety of visceral injuries:

1 *Crush* injuries, where the viscera are injured by pressure against the spine or sacral promontory, by a force applied perpendicularly to the abdomen. In crushing injuries the liver is often lacerated and the duodenum and pancreas are vulnerable.

2 *Tearing* injuries, where the force is applied tangentially to the abdominal wall with the viscera being torn from their peritoneal attachments. Avulsion of the blood supply to the intestinal tract may result and the liver may be torn from the vena cava with consequent severe haemorrhage.

3 *Compression* injuries, where violent compression of the abdomen produces a sudden increased abdominal pressure causing rupture of the gut.

4 *Indirect* injury, can result from (a) the body falling from a height and landing in a vertical position. This frequently results in tearing of the mesentry with subsequent infarction of the gut, or (b) sudden muscular action, such as lifting heavy weights has also been implicated in the rupture of hollow viscera.

The association of bony injury and damage to viscera is most frequently seen in pelvis injuries with associated rupture of the bladder or urethra. Fractures of the lower ribs may be associated with injuries to the liver, spleen or, less frequently, kidney. Evidence of visceral damage is unfortunately variable and difficult to elicit especially in the unconscious patient. Injury to solid viscera causes haemorrhage, whilst injury to the hollow viscera results in peritoneal soiling. In both situations the clinical signs of peritonitis may be present, i.e. abdominal tenderness, resound and diminished or absent bowel sounds. In addition, the general features of shock, such as pallor, sweating, tachycardia and hypotension are frequently seen and indeed may, to a lesser or greater degree result in masking of abdominal signs. In the unconscious patient abdominal signs are also often suppressed.

The basis for suspicion of internal abdominal injury depends on the history, e.g. anatomical site of trauma, pain of increasing severity and extent etc., and also on careful clinical examination which may need to be repeated on a number of occasions. Such repeated examination may demonstrate developing restlessness and pallor, rising pulse rate, falling blood pressure and increasing peritonism, thus suggesting intra-abdominal bleeding. Persisting signs of shock after pain relief and immobilization of fractures strongly suggest intraperitoneal bleeding or peritonitis. Diaphragmatic irritation resulting in referred shoulder tip pain is suggestive of rupture of the spleen or the right lobe of the liver. Bruising and discolouration of the abdominal wall are highly suggestive of severe internal injury, e.g. abrasions of the right hypochondrium might indicate a ruptured liver, abrasions of the left hypochondrium might indicate a ruptured spleen, abrasions in the costolumbar region may indicate renal trauma. Localized swelling suggests local haematoma formation either in the abdominal wall due to rupture of the epigastric artery or to a haematoma in a solid viscus. Generalised abdominal swelling occurring within a few hours of injury is suggestive of severe internal bleeding. Repeated girth measurement is helpful. Percussion may elicit shifting dullness due to haemorrhage, or loss of liver dullness and resonance suggesting perforation. Bowel sounds rapidly disappear following perforation of the intestinal tract but may remain for some hours with haemorrhage. Rectal examination may elicit pelvic swelling suggesting gross peritoneal bleeding or rupture of the urethra.

Radiography is often unhelpful but nevertheless should always be done. Erect and decubitus views of the abdomen may demonstrate free air in the peritoneal cavity; erect films of the abdomen and chest may show elevation of the diaphragm suggesting rupture of the diaphragm or possibly, intrahepatic haematoma. In suspected renal injuries an emergency intravenous pyelogram is often helpful. This will assess injury to an affected kidney and the presence or absence of a contralateral kidney. Arteriography is rarely indicated but aortography should be performed if rupture of the aorta is suspected. Traditional peritoneal 'four-quadrant' tap is an unreliable method of assessing the presence or absence of intraperitoneal bleeding. In contrast, peritoneal lavage with one line of isotonic saline is a highly sensitive method of detecting even small amounts of intra-abdominal haemorrhage, when doubt persists after clinical examination. This procedure, which can be carried out under local anaesthetic, involves the insertion of a dialysis cannula into the peritoneal cavity through a short subumbilical incision. Following infusion of the saline the patient is rolled gently from side to side and the fluid allowed to drain by gravity. Blood staining of the effluent is an indication for laparotomy. When the patient's condition is worse than can be attributed to the obvious injuries or if he fails to respond to adquate resuscitation, then severe concealed bleeding must be suspected. In the unconscious patient, signs of oligomelia again suggests severe haemorrhage.

Liver

The liver is injured most frequently because of its size, its fixity and its proximity to the right lower ribs. The trauma may result in contusion, haematoma formation, subcapsular rupture or separation of a portion. The diagnosis of hepatic rupture can be made quickly, but subcapsular haematomas may be masked and only suspected because of elevation of the right hemidiaphragm. During an operation severe haemorrhage may be controlled temporarily by pressure on the free edge of the lesser omentum, either digitally or by the use of a soft clamp, thus occluding the hepatic artery and the portal vein. Bleeding is stopped by the insertion of mattress sutures which may be tied over absorbable haemostatic packs. Gauze packs may be used at operation but only in extreme circumstances should they be left *in situ*, even in the short term, as they lead to sepsis and possible secondary haemorrhage. Hepatic resection may be required if bleeding cannot be controlled by more conservative measures. Repair of the damaged liver should be followed by careful exploration of the lesser sac to exclude rupture of the duodenum and damage to the body of the pancreas.

Spleen

Splenic rupture frequently occurs after upper abdominal trauma. The bleeding may be primary or delayed. Diagnosis may be difficult and there may be few abdominal signs present. However, the anatomical site of injury and the general features of clinical shock may suggest the diagnosis. Delayed rupture occurs in about 20 per cent of the splenic injuries and may occur days or weeks after the original trauma. Splenic rupture accounts for 15–20 per cent of all cases of severe intra-abdominal bleeding. X-ray may be helpful in showing increased density in the left hypochondrium with elevation of the left side of the diaphragm and displacement of the gastric air bubble and the splenic flexure of the colon. Generally, treatment is splenectomy. However, there has recently been an increasing awareness that a small percentage of patients may develop overwhelming sepsis following splenectomy (the postsplenectomy sepsis syndrome). The pneumococcus organism has been frequently incriminated in this regard. For this reason the possibility of a more conservative surgical approach to the ruptured spleen, e.g. partial resection, implantation of splenic remnants in the greater omentum etc., should now be considered in the appropriate circumstances. When splenectomy is necessary, penicillin should be given in the postoperative period.

Kidney

Much commoner in men than in women, injuries where the kidney is forced backwards or medially against the posterior abdominal wall usually result from compression. Rarely are they associated with severe flexion injuries. The signs of ruptured kidney are haematuria, swelling in the flank due to blood or urine and evidence of concealed bleeding. Emergency IVP usually shows either extravasation of dye into the perirenal tissues or distortion of the calyceal system. Operation is rarely indicated and is most usually carried out to drain a large collection of urine or a perinephric abscess.

Bowel

In bowel rupture the small intestine is involved in 90 per cent of cases, the first three feet of jejunum and the terminal three feet of ileum being most frequently involved. The stomach, duodenum and colon are involved in 10 per cent of cases. The bowel may be contused, ruptured or rendered gangrenous by tearing of the mesentry. Rupture may be complete or incomplete. Incomplete rupture may result in severe haematemesis as in a ruptured gastric mucosa or in melaena where the large bowel mucosa is torn. Complete rupture may be either longitudinal or transverse, situated on either the mesenteric or ant-mesenteric border.

The edges of the rupture are contused and oedematous and the pouting mucosa often prevents the escape of flatus or faeces for some time. Damage to the mesentry of the small bowel, the gastrosplenic ligament or mesocolon with bruising, laceration or detachment occurs in 30–40 per cent of closed intestinal injuries. No one sign is pathognomonic of intestinal rupture. Spreading pain increased by movement, coughing or vomiting, tenderness with guarding and a positive rebound phenomenon occurring within a few hours make operation essential. The decision to 'look and see' rather than 'wait and see' can only be made after repeated examination. Plain films of the abdomen showing free air under the diaphragm is diagnostic of rupture of the gastrointestinal tract; the absence of free air certainly does not exclude intestinal rupture. Contrast films with barium or Raybar are not recommended. Rupture of the stomach is not common and perhaps accounts for 3–4 per cent of all intestinal ruptures. The tear always occurs along the greater curvature. Peritonitis develops rapidly and haematemesis is common with gastric rupture. At operation suture of the ruptured stomach is usually all that is required, although the spleen should be carefully checked. Perforation of the colon occurs in less than 10 per cent of all gut injuries. The fixed ascending and descending colon are most frequently involved and the initial shock is severe. Rapid faecal peritonitis ensues and laparotomy is imperative. Repair or resection of the damaged gut is carried out, together with a defunctioning colostomy and drainage of the abdomen.

Pancreas

Injury to the pancreas occurs in about 4 per cent of all intra-abdominal injuries. It occurs commonly with steering wheel and seat belt trauma. Peritoneal lavage fluid may show high levels of amylase whilst the serum amylase is elevated in only 25 per cent of cases. Diagnosis is difficult and is usually only made at laparotomy. If suspected, prompt exploration, adequate drainage and resection of all devitalised pancreas is necessary. Damage to the pancreas is often followed by prolonged pancreatitis, pancreatic fistula, pseudocyst formation and subphrenic abscess.

Blood vessels

Severe crush injuries are often accompanied by gross retroperitoneal bleeding. The source of the bleeding may be impossible to localise and at laparotomy the posterior peritoneum should not be incised. The shock is often very severe and massive transfusion is often necessary. The inferior and vena cava may be ruptured in association with liver damage but rupture of the aorta is rare. Emergency aortography may be helpful in confirming rupture or integrity of the aorta and demonstrating retroperitoneal haematoma by displacement of adjacent vascular strictures. Occasionally, gross retroperitoneal bleeding may result in a mass palpable per abdomen. Abdominal vascular injuries are dealt with fully in Section III.

Ureters

Ureteric injury is very rare but if it occurs primary repair with or without splinting is the treatment of choice.

In all these traumatic situations the diagnosis is usually obvious within six hours. The other problem facing the general surgeon is the frequent occurrence of paralytic ileus complicating injuries of all kind, acute dilatation of the stomach complicating fractures and paralytic ileus resulting from retroperitoneal haemorrhage and spinal injury. Profuse vomiting, marked abdominal distension and a completely silent abdomen on auscultation make the diagnosis obvious. Treatment is conservative by gastrointestinal suction and intravenous infusion. One must be wary for the infrequent occurrence of early onset mechanical obstruction complicating abdominal trauma in the first ten days after injury.

Penetrating abdominal injuries

Penetrating wounds of the abdomen resulting from stabbing, gun-shots etc., should *all* be explored formally by laparotomy, The track of the foreign body should be followed carefully and all resulting injury to intra-abdominal viscera dealt with in the appropriate manner. Perforations to the gastrointestinal tract may come in pairs. Thus, the lesser sac should always be opened when gastric perforation is present.

Entrance and exit wounds should be excised, debrided and left open for subsequent delayed primary suture.

The importance of repeated examination by the same examiner prior to a decision being made cannot be over-emphasised when abdominal trauma has occurred.

PELVIC INJURY

Injury to the pelvis frequently occurs in road traffic accidents and as the result of crushing injuries. Pelvic fractures can occur as the result of a fall in the elderly person. The pelvis should be routinely X-rayed in:

1 Obvious or suspected pelvic injury.
2 Fracture of the femoral shaft.
3 Multiple injuries.

Classification

Type 1: Fractures with no break in the pelvic ring — stable
Type 2: Fractures with one break in pelvic ring — stable
Type 3: Fractures with two breaks in pelvic ring — unstable
Type 4: Fractures involving the acetabulum.

Treatment

Type 1: e.g. avulsion injury, fracture of wing of ileum or fracture of one public ramus
Type 2: e.g. fracture of two pubic rami on one side.
Both these types are stable, but one must be certain that there has been no damage in the region of the sacro-iliac joint. These patients, even though they have pain, are quite often able to stand. Therefore, bed rest for two, three or four weeks and then re-educate them in walking, initially on crutches, is all that is required.
Type 3: This is an unstable type with two breaks in the ring. These patients are usually in considerable pain, shocked and unable to stand. Three mechanisms of injury have been described.
(a) Anteroposterior compression with fractures of both pubic rami bilaterally giving a central unstable segment in front.
(b) 'Open oyster shell', that is, disruption of the symphysis or fracture of both rami in front, together with dislocation or subluxation of the sacro-iliac joint or fracture close to this joint.
(c) Vertical displacement where the hemipelvis is displaced upwards.
Longitudinal skeletal traction on the affected limb for six to eight weeks may be necessary. Occasionally a plaster of Paris hip spica may be used

and occasionally an external fixator may be required to maintain reduction.

There is usually marked shock and prompt and adequate resuscitation will be needed. Blood transfusion should be started as soon as possible and 10-12 units of blood or even more may be required. Paralytic ileus often occurs and should be treated by conservative measures.

Type 4: Fractures involving the acetabulum, with or without displacement of fragments and perhaps associated with central dislocation of the hip. There may be an indication for surgery to replace a large fragment of acetabulum, particularly if.the weight-bearing surface is involved. Fractures which involve the acetabulum carry with them a risk of subsequent development of osteoarthritis of the hip joint.

Associated soft tissue injury

When injury to the bony pelvis is present the possibility of concomitant soft tissue injury should always be considered. The important organs sometimes injured in pelvic trauma are the urethra and bladder and are usually associated with the unstable type 3 injury.

Rupture of the male urethra — Bulb

The penile urethra is most commonly injured in the region of the bulb by a direct blow as from a kick or the patient falling astride a hard narrow structure. The degree of damage varies considerably. There may be a simple contusion with the mucosa otherwise intact, a hole in the urethral wall of variable size, or complete transection. In severe cases there is always considerable laceration of the corpus spongiosum with extravasation of blood into the surrounding tissues. The haematoma formed in the perineum may be so tense as to embarrass the blood supply to the overlying skin.

Diagnosis

This is usually easy with a history of trauma followed by pain and swelling in the perineum, and blood appearing at the external urethral meatus. There is often retention of urine, but in minor cases the patient may micturate satisfactorily. Indeed, the haematuria may go unnoticed and the incident of trauma be forgotten until months later when the patient appears complaining of difficulty with micturition, having developed a urethral stricture. As a confirmation of diagnosis, an ascending urethrogram will demonstrate the site of injury, and whether or not the urethral wall is intact.

Treatment

Where the patient is able to pass urine freely no active treatment is necessary. As the urethra is potentially infected, a five day course of antibiotics is advisable. Healing is usually rapid and uncomplicated, but it must be remembered that a stricture can develop even after the most trivial injury. A follow-up urethrogram is therefore indicated in all cases to exclude such a complication. If the patient is unable to pass urine spontaneously, it is reasonable to make one attempt at passing a soft catheter, preferably of the silastic type, per urethram. However, as with *any* suspected urethral rupture, repeated attempts to pass a urethral catheter should, *under no circumstances*, take place. When a urethral catheter cannot be inserted, the bladder should be exposed suprapubically and drained with a size 20 catheter of the Foley or silastic type. That done, the question now arises as to whether or not to interfere with the perineal wound. The policy recommended here is a very conservative one; mostly inactivity where the injury is thought to be very mild or moderate as shown by the urethrogram and only a moderate swelling not under tension in the perineum. On the other hand, if the perineal swelling is gross and the skin thinned over it, then the patient is placed in the lithotomy position and the haematoma is evacuated, haemostasis secured as far as possible and the skin closed leaving a small drainage tube in the wound for these days without any attempt at urethral repair.

Both groups are reassessed after ten–fourteen days with a urethrogram and a urethroscopy as necessary. In the majority of the first group an adequate channel can be demonstrated to allow the suprapubic drainage tube to be removed within a month of the injury. Some may require the intermittent passage of dilators. Most of the severe cases will develop a stricture severe enough to warrant operative intervention at a later date. Where there has been minimal interference in the first place, such strictures as do develop can be readily and very successfully repaired. A more aggressive attitude is advocated by some who recommend early exploration of the torn urethra and its immediate repair leaving a small, preferably fenestrated, catheter in the urethra as well as suprapubic drainage. In experienced hands this line of treatment can give excellent results. The inexperienced and junior surgeon is advised to adopt the more conservative approach, leaving the expert to deal with strictures when they arise.

Rupture of the male urethra — membranous

With the ever increasing number of road traffic accidents this is becoming a relatively common problem, particularly in the young adult male. Unlike bladder injury, urethral damage is not infrequently followed by lifelong disability due to stricture, incontinence, impotence and sterility.

Rupture of the urethra must be kept in mind in all cases of fractured pelvis, and the Casualty team of doctors and nurses should be geared to suspect it. The incidence varies between 5 and 25 per cent and approximately 10 per cent of these will have an associated injury to the bladder.

Following crushing or compression of the pelvic girdle the urethra is sheared off at the apex of the prostate on the superficial layer of the urogenital diaphragm. The tear is often partial but may be complete. Haemorrhage is brisk and the local tissues are suffused with blood. The resulting haematoma may displace the prostate and bladder neck well away from its normal position. Extravasation of urine is uncommon. The patient will develop retention due to spasm of the internal sphincter. Too often there are severe associated injuries to the head, chest or abdomen and it is these that demand primary attention.

Diagnosis

Blood appears at the external urethral meatus and may be obvious. Its appearance may be delayed in severely shocked patients and so in suspected cases the Casualty doctor should milk the urethra and record his findings. The patient cannot pass urine. (There is no point in asking him not to attempt to do so). Eventually retention develops, but this may not happen for several hours, depending on the patient's fluid intake and state of shock.

Assessment of the problem

Attention is first directed to a careful evaluation and correction of associated injuries, blood loss and electrolyte imbalance. Secondly attention is directed to the pelvic orthopaedic problem and lastly to the urological problem. Only when the more serious injuries have been dealt with and the patient properly resuscitated, should one attempt to deal with the urethra. Severity of the associated injuries often dictates the type of urological management. There is never any urgency as far as the urethra is concerned. Even when the bladder is also injured, one can afford to wait for twenty-four hours if need be before investigation and treatment is commenced.

Blood at the external meatus, the inability to pass urine with development of retention are proof enough of ruptured urethra but are no guide to the extent of the damage. Rectal examination may reveal displacement of the prostate, but only too often the haematoma at the site of injury so masks the normal anatomy that nothing valuable can be gained by this examination.

An intravenous pyelogram will not only indicate the state of the upper urinary tract, but also of the bladder and whether or not it has been displaced from its normal position in the pelvis. An anterior urethrogram is safe and of value in demonstrating extravasation, but will not always distinguish between a partial and a complete tear. The anterior urethra should be cleansed, the contrast used should be aqueous based and dilute, and the examination ideally carried out with radiological screening.

Treatment

There is considerable controversy as to the best method of treatment and few can speak authoritatively on the subject. These patients often present to the nearest hospital where the individual surgeon's experience of immediate management is small.

Early exploration and immediate repair advocated by some authorities is certainly an attractive concept, but is fraught with considerable difficulties and dangers. Passage of an urethral catheter hoping to get it into the bladder may well succeed, but too often fails and the attempt produces further bleeding and may convert a partial into a complete tear, and introduce infection into the haematoma. At surgical exploration the bladder wall and periprostatic tissues are suffused with blood and there may be active bleeding which is difficult to control. Identification of the torn urethral ends is difficult and further dissection and immobilisation may add to the already existing damaged blood vessels and nerves. The overall results following early operative interference are far from satisfactory with far too high an incidence of stricture, incontinence, impotence and sterility, and it may rightly be suggested that in some cases at least, these bad results are due to unnecessary, or unskilled surgery. Meddlesome surgery initially often makes reconstruction of the urethra later very much more difficult. Therefore the guiding principle advocated is *NOT* to interfere initially with the injured urethra unless there is unquestionable evidence of complete transection with wide displacement of the prostate, and that only when there is an experienced surgeon available to deal with the problem.

Rupture with prostatic displacement

The reported incidence varies greatly from one hospital to another; as low as 5 per cent, and yet as high as 50 per cent. The inexperienced surgeon should simply expose the bladder and under direct vision insert a suprapubic catheter. He may insert the forefinger into the bladder to assess the degree of mobility and displacement of the prostate, but not interfere with the urethra. Inserting the catheter blindly through a stab wound is not recommended.

Management of urethral injury

In many cases of fractured pelvis, management is facilitated by the use of an indwelling urethral catheter. Where the urethra is not injured its use is no problem.

1 Where the patient is very ill as a result of associated injuries and no repair can be considered, a suprapubic cystotomy alone is performed and the bladder is drained with a 24 CH Foley or de Pezzer catheter. The bladder wall should be exposed and the catheter inserted under direct vision. Insertion using blind stab method is not recommended. Urological investigation and treatment may be deferred for a week without detriment to the final result.

2 At the other end of the scale, where the patient's injuries are confined to the pelvis alone, his general state is usually satisfactory, and allows

early assessment and treatment, or where the shocked patient has been quickly and adequately resuscitated

(a) With no obvious prostatic displacement a simple suprapubic cystotomy is performed and a drain placed into the retropubic space. This drain allows the extravasated blood to escape and promotes early resolution at the site of rupture. After three weeks the state of the urethra can be assessed with urethrogram and urethroscopy. In the majority of cases the urethra will have healed, so that the suprapubic drain can be removed.

(b) With wide prostatic displacement, the inexperienced surgeon would do well to perform a suprapubic cystotomy only and transfer the patient to a Urological Department. The experienced operator will explore the retropubic space, carefully remove the haematoma, secure haemostasis, which can be difficult, define the torn ends of the urethra and pass a 20 CH Foley catheter along the anterior urethra and guide it into the bladder. Great care is taken to ensure that the torn ends of the proximal urethra are not inverted during the introduction of the catheter. The aim is to achieve a proper realigment of the torn urethra and to maintain it in the correct position. The author uses a few 2XO catgut sutures placed through the apex of the prostate and the puboprostatic ligaments. They are not passed through the urethral mucosa. Traction on the indwelling urethral catheter is not recommended.

3 Where the patient is already in the operating theatre undergoing an emergency operation for other serious injuries and there has been no time for urological assessment

(a) The inexperienced surgeon should perform a suprapubic cystotomy only.

(b) The expert surgeon will open the bladder and with the forefinger at the internal urethral meatus, can assess whether or not the prostate is mobile and displaced. If there is no obvious displacement, then a suprapubic catheter is inserted and the retropubic space drained. If the urethral tear is complete then he should proceed to immediate repair as described.

Rupture of the female urethra

The female urethra is short and not often exposed to the same traumatic forces as in the male. Rupture may occur in fracture of the pelvis, and is usually incomplete and can be adequately managed with an indwelling urethral catheter in minor cases. Suprapubic bladder drainage is advised where there is an expensive periurethral haematoma. Stricture is a rare complication.

Rupture of the bladder

Injuries to the bladder occur most commonly in male adults and are rare at the extremes of age. Bladder injury alone is seldom serious. Less than one per cent of patients with major trauma sustained in road traffic accidents die as a result of their pelvic injuries.

Open injuries

Open injuries caused by gunshot or stabbing are rarely uncomplicated and are often associated with injury to the colon or rectum and are therefore usually infected. The extent of injury to the bladder varies greatly and may be very small and the patient able to pass urine afterwards. Indeed the author has seen a young soldier pass per urethra a bullet which had entered his bladder through the perineum and rectum. With high velocity bullets there is considerable destruction of tissue along its path. After preliminary resuscitation these wounds must be carefully explored, requiring intraperitoneal as well as perivesical and intravesical inspection. Wounds of the vault are easily excised and repaired. Those of the bladder base may be difficult to define and difficult to repair. In these the bladder is best drained by a suprapubic catheter, with drainage of the perivesical space, and, where the rectum is also involved, a proximal defunctioning colostomy is performed. With these methods the bladder and rectum will usually heal without fistula formation.

Closed injuries

These may be intraperitoneal or extraperitoneal, the latter being more common in proportion of six to one.

1 Intraperitoneal rupture

This occurs only when the bladder is fully distended, following a heavy blow to the lower abdomen, or a run-over accident. The bladder literally bursts. The tear in the superoposterior wall is usually large with free escape of urine into the peritoneal cavity. This initial flooding of the peritoneum is not in any way serious as the urine is sterile. Many of the patients are under the influence of alcohol at the time of their accident and diagnosis may be difficult and delayed.

Diagnosis. There may be local bruising and rigidity over the bladder area and the patient will not pass urine, peritoneal irritation from the extravasated urine is slight and initially the patient's general condition is very good when the bladder alone is injured. Gradually the abdomen becomes distended with absence of bowel sounds. In some, shoulder tip pain may suggest the diagnosis. Intraperitoneal rupture is rarely associated with ruptured urethra.

Pre-Operative Investigation. Confirmation of the diagnosis is made by intravenous pyelogram, which will not only demonstrate the rupture, but also the integrity, or otherwise, of the upper urinary tract. Double injuries of the renal tract are not uncommon. If there is no blood at the external urethral meatus, an ascending urethrogram and cystogram is a reasonable alternative. An abdominal tap may be unrewarding.

Treatment. The bladder is explored through a mid-line suprapubic incision, allowing firstly detailed inspection of the gastrointestinal tract. The extravasated fluid is removed by suction and the bladder tear is defined, its edges are trimmed and the interior of the bladder inspected, and repair can be carried out in two layers with 2XO chromic sutures. In uncomplicated cases the peritoneal cavity is closed without drainage and the bladder drained with an indwelling urethral catheter for seven days. Drainage of the retropubic space is only indicated if there has been delay in diagnosis and/or suspicion of local infection. In the rare event of an associated injury to the urethra, then the bladder is drained by a suprapubic catheter, and no catheter in the urethra.

2   Extraperitoneal rupture

This is often associated with fracture of the pelvic girdle when a specule of bone penetrates the bladder wall. The wound in the bladder is usually small and extravasation slight. The patient may be able to pass urine successfully. There may be an associated injury to the posterior urethra in roughly 10 per cent of cases.

Diagnosis. Early diagnosis is not always easy. Local bruising and tenderness may mask the lesion. An IVP is desirable but may not demonstrate the rupture and where a bladder lesion alone is suspected then an ascending urethrogram and cystogram may be necessary.

Treatment. The bladder is exposed and inspected. There may be considerable effusion of blood into the bladder wall and perivesical tissues, making identification of the tear difficult. Where this can be easily visualised it is repaired in two layers, but, if inaccessible, the bladder is opened and inspected from within. If the tear is small it can be left without suturing and the bladder drained with a suprapubic catheter for ten days. A small drain is left down to the site of injury for three days.

Prognosis. The bladder has a very good blood supply and in all types of injury heals satisfactorily after careful repair and adequate drainage. It quickly returns to normal volume and function and without late complications.

THORACOLUMBAR SPINAL INJURIES

The most vulnerable area of the thoracolumbar spine is the thoraco-lumbar junction from the 10th thoracic vertebrae to the 2nd lumbar vertebrae. It is vulnerable to injury at this point because the fixed thoracic spine joins the lumbar spine at this point.

The same basic principles as described for the cervical spine must be applied to suspected injuries at this level. Flexion-rotational forces applied to this area can produce very unstable injuries where the spinal cord is at considerable risk. If the possibility of a spinal injury exists at this level then the usual careful neurological assessment is required and the spine must also be carefully examined. By cautious 'log rolling', whilst applying longitudinal traction to the body, the patient may be turned on to ones side to expose the back. Inspection will often reveal signs of unilateral trauma to the shoulders or ribs and this indicates asymmetrical force having been applied to the body and should increase the examiner's suspicions that rotation has occurred with the effect of increasing spinal instability. Careful palpation of the spinous processes may reveal a discrete area of tenderness. Tearing of the interspinous ligaments with an acute kyphus due to anterior collapse results in the examiner being able to palpate a prominent spinous process and below it, the finger will be able to enter into a gap between the spinous processes. Together these two signs are pathognomonic of an unstable spinal injury.

Trauma at this level is often associated with serious intra-abdominal or intrathoracic injuries which may well be life-threatening and require immediate treatment. If the patient is to be moved from one hospital to another then a firm stretcher should be used and slight hyperextension of the spine will help to hold the spine in a more stable position. This can be achieved by simply placing a pillow under the patient at the appropriate level. The same can be done on the operating table if chest or abdominal surgery is necessary.

In the presence of neurological damage, dexamethasone should be administered in large doses and consideration given to early open reduction and internal fixation of the spine to relieve cord pressure and ensure stability. This is best achieved with Harrington rod fixation. In the patient without nerve involvement, careful thought should also be given to ensuring that all unstable injuries are treated by adequate immobili-sation or internal fixation as serious complications may arise at a later date due to chronic subluxation of the spine.

A significant number of stable injuries will be seen, e.g. the wedge compression fracture, the burst fracture which may be associated with neurological damage and fractures of the vertebral appendages. The majority of these may be treated expectantly with early mobilisation.

LIMB INJURIES

It is best to keep in mind a simple classification of limb injuries:
  Lacerations
    Simple
    Over bones
    Over joints
  Ligamentous/Capsular Injury
    Sprain
    Ruptured Ligaments
    Dislocation/Subluxation
  Vascular Injury
  Fractures
  Muscle/tendon injury
  Nerve injury

After all clothing has been removed all four limbs must be inspected for lacerations, gross deformity, swelling, bruising, unusual attitude of a limb, loss of function and pallor or cyanosis. All four limbs must be palpated from the shoulders to the fingers and from the hips to the toes. A note is made of tenderness, palpable deformity, instability in the region of long bones, unusual instability at joints, coolness, deficient or absent peripheral pulses, loss of sensation and motor power. It is important to record all abnormal findings in the patient's chart.

Lacerations after inspection must be temporarily covered with a sterile dressing. As soon as possible these should be cleansed and redressed with or without sutures. Clean wounds may be sutured. Dirty wounds must be cleansed and all devitalised tissue radically excised until only clean healthy tissue remains. Primary suture should not be carried out but instead delayed wound closure several days later either by sutute or skin graft. Dirty lacerations which are not sufficiently debrided become infected. This is a serious complication and of course is even more serious if the laceration overlies and is in communication with an underlying fracture. A fracture with an overlying laceration of the soft tissues is referred to as an open or compound fracture. This is dealt with more fully in Section III. A laceration overlying and communicating with a joint interior is referred to as an open joint injury and is considered serious and again must be cleansed carefully and debrided. The interior of the joint must be inspected for foreign material and if found, removed. Tetanus prophylaxis and antibiotics should be instituted and these are dealt with in more detail later in this section.

A sprain is an injury to a ligament where only several fibres are ruptured but the integrity of the ligament as a whole remains intact. There is no mechanical instability but there may be tenderness and swelling over the ligament. These should be treated symptomatically.

However, even in the presence of a normal appearing X-ray significant ligamentous damage may have occurred at a joint particularly at the knee and at the ankle joint. A high index of suspicion should be aroused by tenderness, swelling with or without bruising around joints with regard to ligamentous rupture. Tests for stability should be carried out on the affected joints and if difficult to perform, one should consider general anaesthesia in order to assess more properly. X-rays taken of joints whilst various stresses are applied are often useful. Gross deformity at a joint or an unusual attitude of a limb may indicate a dislocation of a joint. The area should be evaluated further by X-ray as soon as possible. Common joint dislocations involve the shoulder, elbow, ankle and less commonly the hip. These should be reduced as soon as possible under general anaesthesia and then immobilised by traction, strapping, Plaster of Paris cast or sling as the case dictates.

A pulseless, cool limb indicates serious arterial injury until proven otherwise. Arterial damage when it occurs is often associated with a fracture or dislocation. Once arterial injury is suspected the artery must be assessed by either an arteriogram or by surgical exploration. Where there is strong suspicion of arterial damage it is best to explore the artery surgically as soon as possible as this will save valuable time. Vascular injury of the limbs is dealt with more fully in Section 3.

Fractured bones with gross deformity should have the deformity reduced by longitudinal traction applied gently to the limb. A temporary splint, e.g. a Thomas splint, for a fractured shaft of femur should be applied to prevent redisplacement of the fracture and for the comfort of the patient. In fractures of the upper limb a sling may be sufficient but very unstable fractures may require a Plaster of Paris backslab. Sedation may be necessary in order that these manipulations can be carried out. Further evaluation by X-ray at the appropriate time is necessary for the proper assessment. These X-rays should include the adjacent joints of the fractured bone.

Lacerated or ruptured tendons as a result of injury are detected by the appropriate loss of function and should be repaired primarily as soon as possible. Muscle ruptures, unless complete and involving an important muscle are generally not surgically repaired.

All injured limbs must have their neurological status assessed. Peripheral nerve injury varies from mild to severe. If it is mild and no more than a concussion of the nerve which will recover in a few days it is referred to as a neuropraxia. Axonotmesis is the term applied to more serious injury of the nerve in which the enveloping sheath is still intact but the nerve has been damaged and will degenerate from the point of injury distally. This condition will recover and the axon will regenerate at approximately one millimetre per day. During the period of recovery it is important to keep the affected joints and muscles supple. These should be passed through a full range of passive motion daily. Splints to prevent contractures may be necessary. The term neurotmesis indicates that the nerve has been completely severed and nothing less than a surgical repair will procure optimal recovery. Another type of serious nerve injury is caused by stretching. This often results in intraneural scarring and a poor recovery is often the result. Most neurological deficits associated with closed injuries are treated expectantly for several weeks or months. Electrical studies can be carried out at a later stage on the affected nerves and these can be very useful in helping to decide whether nerve improvement is occurring or not. Usually after about two months, nerves which are not severed begin to show some recovery at least on electrical studies. However, if after two months, there is still no sign of improvement in the neurological status with regard to peripheral nerve, this nerve should be explored. If a skin wound overlies the course of a nerve the wound should be explored to establish whether the nerve has or has not been divided. Clinical assessment, particularly in children, is often inadequate. If the nerve has been cleanly divided, completely or partially, repair using fine instruments and fine suture material is appropriate, with careful attention to the orientation of the nerve ends. Some magnification is highly desirable. Where there has been significant crushing of the nerve it should be left unrepaired, and re-explored some weeks later.

Of all the injuries to the limbs, vascular injury is the most urgent requiring immediate assessment and definitive treatment if serious impairment to limb function, or indeed, loss of the limb itself is to be prevented. Next comes open fractures which require debridement in order to reduce the risk of infection. Next as a matter of urgency comes dislocated joints which should be reduced as soon as possible to relieve pain and minimize the risk of secondary complications.

3 Drug treatment

The seriously injured patient may require analgesia, antibiotics, anti-tetanus prophylaxis and occasionally an anxiolytic, anti-epileptic and steroids.

Analgesia

If a seriously injured patient is conscious and in pain the pain should be relieved. Severe pain increases anxiety and apprehension and by releasing catecholamines causes vasoconstriction, sweating and tachycardia and so can mimic haemorrhage. Tissue perfusion will be improved by relieving pain. If breathing is shallow because of the severe pain of fractured ribs, oxygenation will be improved by relieving the pain and allowing the injured patient to breathe more freely.

Before any analgesia is given, however, the injured patient must be examined and his clinical condition and his injuries and their severity recorded. If there are limb fractures they should be splinted and well applied splints are immediately effective in relieving pain. Gentle handling and reassurance at all times will also minimise pain. The analgesia chosen must be one that is effective but as safe as possible, and its dose should be one that will relieve the pain. The two types of analgesia that can be used in the early management of the injured patient are inhalation and parenteral.

Inhalation analgesia

Nitrous oxide, given as Entonox, which is 50 per cent nitrous oxide and 50 per cent oxygen, is the most commonly used inhalation analgesic, and it is carried in every ambulance. It is a very effective analgesic, free from serious depressant and unwanted side effects on respiration and circulation, and maximal pain relief is achieved in about two minutes. Complete recovery, without any residual analgesia, occurs in the same time, so it does not mask injuries.

The cylinder is connected to a demand inhalation unit and the demand valve is incorporated in the hand piece. It is normally administered by the patient himself and can be supervised by non-medical personnel. If the injured patient is unable to cooperate, e.g. owing to arm fractures, the mask can be held to his face. If he is unable to breathe deeply the demand valve can be overridden by a press button control and the gases released under positive pressure, but this removes the safeguards conferred by self-administration. Entonox can be offered to almost all the injured who are in pain but should not be administered to those whose consciousness is impaired due to a head injury or intoxication. Those with facio-maxillary injuries are unlikely to be able to tolerate the mask and it should not be given to a patient known to have a pneumothorax as the nitreous oxide passes rapidly into the air pocket.

Entonox is very useful and safe for pain relief at the site of the accident and on the way to hospital when a doctor may not be present. It is very helpful when fractures are being splinted, either at the accident site or in the Accident and Emergency Department, and it is excellent when a fracture-dislocation has to be reduced without delay, e.g. at the ankle where the circulation could be impaired. There are two precautions which must be taken when using Entonox at the site of an accident. The first is because of its 50 per cent oxygen content which necessitates that it must be used with the same care as pure oxygen when cutting equipment is being used. The second must be remembered when working in very cold conditions. Below – 6 degrees centigrade nitreous oxide tends to liquefy and fall to the bottom of the cylinder so that at first pure oxygen will be inhaled but later pure nitreous oxide. The cylinder should not be stored in a very cold area and if there is any doubt it must be turned upside down to mix the gases.

Parenteral analgesia

A seriously injured patient is very likely to be shocked with vasoconstriction of muscle and subcutaneous tissues, therefore any analgesic given by one of these routes will be very poorly absorbed with little or no pain relief. A second injection may be given and when tissue perfusion is improved there will be a cumulative effect. All parenteral agents should therefore be given intravenously, in small incremental doses until the desired effect is reached.

The most effective analgesia is morphia. It almost always gives pain relief and mental sedation if the dose is sufficient. It has disadvantages, however, and these are sometimes feared so much that it is withheld from the injured patient, allowing pain to increase distress and shock. What are the disadvantages of morphia, and how can they be overcome?

1 It may depress laryngeal reflexes, respiration and circulation and this depression is accentuated in patients with respiratory embarrassment due to chest injury or decreased cardiac output due to haemorrhage or pump

failure. It must therefore be used with caution in seriously ill patients. As a shocked patient may be very sensitive to even a small dose of morphia it is wise to start an intravenous infusion and administer oxygen before giving morphia and the first increment should be half the normal dose. The depressant effect is usually decreased in the presence of severe pain, however, and further increments may be required but must be given slowly and cautiously. A patient with a chest injury that is causing severe pain should not be denied morphia, as the pain relief may improve his clinical condition. His ventilation must be watched carefully, however, and if the morphia is thought to be depressing respiration it can be reversed by giving naloxone (Narcan) intravenously.

2 It constricts the pupils and a severe head injury is said to be an absolute contra-indication to its use, but a patient with a severe head injury is usually unconscious and does not require analgesia. If a patient with a slight head injury is in severe pain due to trauma elsewhere, morphia should not be denied.

Severe headache in the early post-traumatic phase should always raise the suspicion of a complication, but analgesia need not be withheld. A small dose of morphia can be given but the nurse who is observing the patient must be told to report any lowering of the level of consciousness immediately and not assume it is due to the analgesia. If there is any cause for concern the effect of the morphia can be reversed by intravenous Narcan.

3 Nausea and vomiting are not often seen in the presence of severe pain, but cyclizine (Valoid) can be given with the morphia or in combination as Cyclimorph.

4 Its effect lasts 1–2 hours and may create diagnostic difficulties. The patient's clinical condition must be carefully assessed and recorded prior to giving morphia and if he deteriorates the pain relief can be temporarily reversed if necessary by Narcan.

Morphia should be given in a dose that will relieve pain and a fit adult in severe pain may require 20–40 mg but this will be given slowly in increments.

Antibiotics

The question of prophylactic antibiotics is a vexed one and the trend is away from giving them routinely in trauma. Soft tissue injuries are much better protected from infection by thorough surgical toilet and if necessary delayed primary suture than by antibiotics. An exception may be a deep penetrating injury where good surgical toilet is not possible, and ampicillin/flucloxicillin (Magnapen) is popular at the moment.

Even with a compound fracture of the skull and a CSF leak some neurosurgeons do not give prophylactic antibiotics unless the wound is exceptionally dirty. Others do and the choice of drug is personal but Magnapen 500 mg and Sulphadimidine GLIM stat (adult) is often used. Orthopaedic surgeons often give a stat. dose of Magnapen 500 mg IM to patients with compound fractures unless they are known to be allergic to penicillin when erythromycin can be used. If there is an open abdominal wound gentamycin 80 mg IM and metranidazole (Flagyl) 500 mg in 100 mg IV stat. is recommended.

Anti-tetanus prophylaxis

All wounds, no matter how trivial, are susceptible to tetanus, and surgical toilet is of prime importance. Immunity must be ensured and the scheme

All wounds receive surgical toilet

Wounds that are less than six hours old. Clean. Non-penetrating and with negligible tissue damage.		Other wounds	
Immunity category	*Treatment*	*Immunity category*	*Treatment*
A	Nothing more required	A	Nothing more required
B	Toxoid 1 dose	B	Toxoid 1 dose
C	Toxoid 1 dose	C	Toxoid 1 dose and human tetanus immunoglobulin
D	Toxoid complete course	D	Toxoid complete course and human tetanus immunoglobulin

A has had a complete course of toxoid or a booster dose within the past five years.
B has had a complete course of toxoid or a booster dose more than five and less than ten years ago.
C has had a complete course of toxoid or a booster dose more than ten years ago.
D has not had a complete course of toxoid or immunity status is unknown.

recommended by Smith, Laurence and Evans (BMJ 23rd August 1975) is the one that is usually followed. It should be remembered that a natural attack of tetanus does not produce immunity. Tetanus toxoid (0.5 ml) and human tetanus immunoglobulin 250 units (Humotet) must not be given into the same limb. Adrenaline injection (BP) should be available during prophylactic procedures for the treatment of anaphylactic shock (in adults 0.5–1 ml IM) but a severe reaction is extremely unlikely to occur in a previously healthy patient. The use of antibiotics is not included in the scheme as the authors believe that with the availability of Humotet they should now mainly revert to their role of dealing with sepsis.

Reactions to aluminium adsorbed toxoid are rare and usually no more than pain and swelling at the injection site. If a patient has reacted to a previous injection 0.1 ml of non-adsorbed simple toxoid can be given intradermally. Fluid toxoid is less reactogenic than adsorbed toxoid but is also less antigenic (Dick G (1974) *Update* 8, 1011).

Anxiolytic

If a severely injured patient is very anxious and shaking with fear a small dose of diazepam (Valium) given very slowly intravenously can improve his condition and make him more cooperative, but before giving it make sure that the anxiety is not due to hypoxia.

Anti-epileptic

If a patient with a head injury has fits they must be controlled and diazepam given by slow intravenous injection in a dose sufficient to stop the fits is the drug most commonly used.

Steroids

Steroids have not been proven to be of any value in traumatic shock or acute head injury. A stat. dose of 30 mg Dexamethazone IV is often recommended for a patient with a fracture-dislocation of the cervical spine and paralysis.

Summary

Treatment of the severely injured patient

Analgesia	Entonox or Morphia
Antibiotics	In some cases
Antitetanus prophylaxis	A must
Anxiolytic	Rarely
Antiepileptic	If needed
Steroids	Rarely

4 Mobilisation of staff

It is most important to ask yourself the question 'should I be calling for help?'. It is easy to get so deeply involved in other aspects that you forget this. Especially when two or three patients arrive simultaneously, you should think of calling extra doctors, for although you start with the patient who appears the most serious, he may not be the most serious. If matters look very grave, do not hesitate to call for very senior colleagues. Colleagues may be needed regarding a patient with multiple injuries to decide whether all injuries will be dealt with in one operation, or in stages, and which ward the patient should go to. Sometimes the injuries are the responsibility of one speciality. Remember to contact that ward and the theatre so that when resuscitation is complete, no unnecessary delay occurs.

5   Making a good record

This must be done immediately, Often the patient will pass from the care of one team to another. It is most important that there is full record of everything found at examination, all investigations ordered and all treatment which has been carried out. It is very difficult in the highly charged emotional atmosphere to remember things accurately even for a few minutes. If possible, one person should do the examination, dictating his findings while he is actually looking and feeling. A second person writes down the record as it is dictated. These six aspects have had to be written down one after the other, but in practice all six have to proceed each interwoven with the other. It is possible nevertheless to have a clear picture in the mind, of what must be achieved and to end up with a well resuscitated patient, a good record and colleagues on good terms with each other.

6 Monitoring the patient's condition

Time passes very quickly as one is absorbed in resuscitation and examining. It is important to know whether the patient is getting better or worse. In order that this may be gauged, a nurse must be detailed to take clinical observations of pulse and respiration rates, blood pressure, the pupil reactions, the word responsiveness and movement responsiveness of the patient. The doctor must see that these are being recorded and must look at the record from time to time to assess its meaning. Central venous pressure readings and urine output may be helpful. A number of laboratory tests may establish a baseline which will be useful in further monitoring. These include haemoglobin, haematocrit, urea and electrolytes, blood gases and blood alcohol.

A certain proportion of these patients will require more intensive observation and treatment. These facilities are available in a modern intensive care unit. These patients have potentially life-threatening injuries. Therefore, minute to minute observation of the vital functions of respiration, cardiovascular haemodynamics, central nervous system and renal function is essential. Frequent estimations of acid base, blood gases and blood sugars are also required. The collective term for this is *monitoring* from the Latin word — *monere* — to warn. Early types of monitor include the stethoscope, clinical thermometer and sphygomomanometer. The best monitor is a highly skilled and experienced nurse in constant attendance but this is not always possible. Obviously some signals cannot be measured and recorded directly by nurses nor can they record continuously or at very frequent intervals. Initially, some thought was given to the problem of how one nurse could look after several patients. The development of the oscilloscope led to bedside monitoring and central consoles. In 1962, Hughes Day in the Bethany Hospital, Kansas City, reported on the continuous monitoring of patients with myocardial infarcts in a Coronary Care Unit. In 1962, the mortality was 19 per cent as against 39 per cent in 1961. Before discussing the various systems and what can be monitored, remember there is no monitor that will tell us the colour of the patient and what his response to stimuli is. The same applies to the level of consciousness and the degree of abdominal distension. Thus, monitors are not going to replace the clinician.

A transducer converts physiological pressures to electrical signals, e.g. a catheter in an artery with the pressure transmitted to a flushing dome and then to a flexible pressure sensitive diaphragm. The movement of the diaphragm is directly proportional to the pressure in the vessel. This is then relayed to a calibrated meter for display.

Respiration

Automated self-calibrating blood gas analysis machines enables measurements of PO^2, PCO^2 and pH to be performed rapidly and accurately. These measurements are essential in the management of the traumatised patient, especially when respiratory inadequacy occurs. Newer techniques such as intravascular polargraphic electrodes are still under trial but continuous display of blood gases would be a major advance. Transcutaneous techniques of monitoring PO^2 have proved disappointing as they are inaccurate in the presence of peripheral vasoconstriction and hypothermia.

If respiration is inadequate some form of mechanical support is required. Respiration may be assisted or completely controlled. The tidal volume, respiratiory rate and inspired oxygen concentration are preselected and adjusted according to the patient's needs.

Apnoea alarms

They are incorporated in most modern ventilators but are also available for the spontaneously breathing patients. End tidal CO^2 can be monitored using a capnometer and provides instantaneous information in changes in end tidal CO^2 and has the advantage of being non-invasive.

Oxygen analysers

It is mandatory to be able to check and adjust the inspired oxygen concentration on any patient receiving oxygen therapy because of the dangers of pulmonary oxygen toxicity. Oxygen analysers are incorporated into the ventilator or may be available as a separate item of equipment.

Cardiovascular haemodynamics

Ninety per cent of patients who are hypotensive are usually hypovolaemic and respond to blood, albumin and crystalloid. Occasionally inotropic agents such as dopamine and dobutamine are required. Potent drugs must be carefully infused intravenously in the correct dilution over a prolonged period. The introduction of accurate volume counters has simplified their adminstration and increased the patient's safety. The syringe pump, especially, allows very small volumes to be infused.

Electrocardiograph (ECG)

It is the most commonly used monitor in wards, intensive care units and operating rooms. Indeed, it may be considered medico-legally negligent to omit this early warning system in the case of critically ill patients. We are interested in heart rate, arrhythmias and changes in the T-wave.

Pulse monitors

They are sometimes used and only record the heart rate. They respond to changes in light and incorporate a photo-electric cell.

Blood pressure

There are many methods including cuff, palpation, oscillometer and microphone used to amplify the sounds. Ultrasound detects movements of the vessel wall. Invasive techniques with insertion of a catheter into a peripheral artery such as the radial or dorsalis pedis and connected via a transducer to a screen for display are the most accurate and useful.

Central venous pressure (CVP)

This is measured from the tip of a catheter placed in a central vein and can be measured by simple displacement of a water column or connected via a transducer to a screen. This pressure provides a useful relationship between blood returning to the right atrium and the ability of the right ventricle to pump it into the pulmonary circulation. It can be helpful in detecting and treating hypovolaemia and diagnosing right heart failure.

Cardiac output

The development and clinical application of the pulmonary artery catheter (Swan–Ganz) has made possible the bedside monitoring of cardiac output using the principle of thermodilution with a thermistor capable of detecting small changes in temperature. The cardiac output can be calculated knowing the amount of cold fluid injected and the time duration and magnitude of the temperature changes. The advantage of this technique enables repeated measurements to be made.

Swan-Ganz cathether

This is a flotation catheter which can be wedged in the pulmonary artery. The wedge pressure is similar to the left atrial pressure and thus information about the left side of the heart can be derived indirectly. Hypovolaemia in the presence of a normal or elevated CVP can be detected as well as left heart failure.

Central nervous system

Intracranial pressure is by far the most useful form of measurement monitored in the severe head injury patient. It is not only a guide to the severity of the injury but it is essential if the proper treatment is to be instituted. It is also helpful engaging progress. A sensor is inserted through a burr hole in the skull and placed under the dura mater. The resulting pressure is displayed in digital form.

Temperature

Although the mercury glass thermometer is still in use, the simultaneous measurement of skin, oesophageal and rectal temperature with suitable probes allows temperature monitoring to be more precise and informative.

Fat embolism

This is a syndrome occasionally associated with fractures and in particular fractures of the shaft of the femur. Petechiae may be seen on the chest wall and in the axillae. Respiratory insufficiency may develop, and if it does, it may require respiratory assistance. Fat embolism can be fatal.

Section 2
Injury to specific parts

7   The eye, eyelid and orbit

The eye and its adnexae are highly specialised tissues which respond unfavourably to trauma. Even mild scarring may adversely affect the optical properties of the eye with dire consequences for vision. It is axiomatic that in repair of eye injuries medial clarity should be preserved and intra-ocular organization kept to a mininum. Most eye injuries require the attention of an ophthalmic surgeon with access to specialised equipment and where multiple injuries are present the eye should be protected with a resilient periorbital shield until appropriate treatment can be instituted.

The evaluation of ocular and adnexal injuries should include a detailed history of the event with particular reference to foreign bodies, evaluation of visual functions and examination of the eyes, both anterior and posterior segments, under magnification.

Eyelid injuries

Superficial lacerations

Most superficial lacerations can be satisfactorily sutured under local anaesthetic using either 6/0 silk or 6/0 nylon. Eyelid skin is thin with relatively little subcutaneous fat and a mattress suture is often required to prevent inversion of the skin edges.

Deep, full-thickness eyelid lacerations

Deep lacerations may involve full-thickness eyelid and orbital septum with prolapse of orbital fat. The underlying globe may also be perforated in which instance there will be loss of vision, hypotonia of the globe and vitreous haemorrhage. During major repairs of upper or lower eyelids the eye itself must be protected, usually with a scleral contact lens. Imperfectly repaired eyelid lacerations cause long-term ocular discomfort and occasionally ocular scarring with loss of vision. Ideally, all eyelid lacerations should be sutured by an ophthalmic or plastic surgeon and it is better to delay surgical repair of an eyelid rather than execute imperfect apposition or repair of tissues. Perforation of the orbital septum should be closed with 5/0 or 6/0 catgut after repositioning orbital fat. Tarsal plate lacerations and orbicularis muscle defects should be carefully aligned and sutured with 5/0 catgut. Skin closure should be effected with 6/0 silk or nylon. Lacerations involving the tendenous expansion of levator palpebrae superiorus may cause ptosis and if large should be carefully exposed and meticulously sutured with 5/0 chromic catgut.

Laceration involving eyelid margins

Marginal lacerations must be meticulously apposed to prevent lid notching, trichiasis and keratotic plaque formation which cause irritation and scarring of the cornea. Lid wounds should be carefully cleaned and trimmed and the sharp apposing edges then precisely closed in three layers. The lid margin should be aligned using two 6/0 silk sutures, one placed and the level of the grey line and the other just posterior to the lash line. The tarsal plate edges are accuragely apposed with 5/0 or 6/0 chromic catgut sutures and orbicularis oculae with 6/0 plain catgut. The skin is closed with 6/0 silk or nylon.

All secondary repairs of the upper or lower eyelids are the preserve of an experienced ophthalmic or plastic surgeon.

Eyelid lacerations with tissue loss — eyelid avulsion

Prior to repair, the anterior segment of the eye must be protected with moist saline swabs or scleral contact lens. Immediate surgery and repair is directly towards achieving adequate protection of the eyelid. Careful repair of the various eyelid components is undertaken under a dry field and defects closed by mobilizing, transferring or transplanting eyelid or facial tissue. Extensive reconstructive surgery may be required at a later date.

Burns

Superficial eyelid burns are caused by electric arc flashes, ultraviolet lights and industrial detergents. Most heal quickly and require only careful cleaning and removal of residual chemical particles or foreign bodies. The cornea and conjuctiva may be involved and antibiotic and cycloplegic drops should be instilled to control the underlying keratitis and conjunctivitis.

Deep burns are usually a consequence of splashing the eyelids with acid or alkali or occur as part of a generalised facial burn. If severe necrosis is present early grafting may be required to prevent scarring, contracture and loss of eyelid function.

Injuries to the conjunctiva

Contusion, haemorrhage, chemosis

Subjunctival haemorrhages resolve within two or three weeks and require no treatment. Occasionally a dense subjunctival haemorrhage may camouflage an underlying scleral rupture or indicate a fracture at the base of the skull or orbital bones. Loss of vision, vitreous haemorrhage and abnormally low intraocular pressure indicate the presence of a scleral tear or rupture. The patient should be immediately prepared for exploration of the globe under general anaesthesia.

Lacerations

All conjunctival lacerations should be explored to exclude an underlying perforating scleral wound. Small uncomplicated conjunctival lacerations may be left unsutured if the wound margins are approximated and no Tenon's capsule is protruding. Extensive conjunctival lacerations should be sutured using 6/0 plain catgut. Any associated scleral or extra-ocular muscle laceration should be carefully sutured using an operating microscope.

Foreign bodies

Conjunctival foreign bodies are common and characteristically lodge in the subtarsal sulcus beneath the upper eyelid. Small foreign bodies can be removed using a cotton tip applicator after a thorough search of the fornices and after everting the upper eyelid. Multiple loose foreign bodies or particulate chemical matter can be removed by irrigating the conjunctival sac with normal saline. Foreign bodies that have become embedded in the interpalpebral conjunctiva following blast injuries should be teased free with a needle or fine forcep, otherwise unsightly tattoo marks will persist.

Burns

Chemical burns of the conjunctiva are ocular emergencies and usually involve the anterior segment of the eye. Alkali rapidly penetrate the cornea and cause a severe inflammatory reaction in the anterior chamber and irreversible damage to the anterior uvea. Immediate and meticulous irrigation of the conjunctival sac is required with removal of all particulate chemical material. Chelating agents may be useful in lime burns and antibiotic drops should be prescribed to prevent secondary infection. Collagenase inhibitors (acetyl cysteine) and local or systemic steroids may be required to preserve integrity of the conjunctiva and cornea and suppress intra-ocular inflammation. Conjunctival adhesions may develop and should be relieved using a glass rod lubricated with antibiotic ointment. Maintenance of the fornices may require insertion of a scleral contact lens for a period of time.

Injuries to the eye

Corneal abrasion

The extent of the abrasion may be determined using a fluorescein drop. After instillation of a local anaesthetic drop (Amethocaine 1 per cent) into the conjuctival sac, all foreign bodies should be removed and a short acting mydriatic and cycloplegic instilled to relieve spasm of the ciliary muscle. A firm pad and bandage is applied to prevent excessive eye movement over the lesion. The patient should be referred to an ophthalmic outpatient clinic to document and confirm healing of the abrasion. Local anaesthetic drops should be used for diagnostic purposes only and have no part in any therapeutic regimen.

Corneal foreign body

Superficial corneal foreign bodies can be removed using a moistened cotton tip applicator or superficially embedded foreign bodies may be removed with a sharp pointed instrument or needle under direct vision aided by slit lamp biomicroscopy. Rust rings which contain ferrous particles and irritate the cornea should be meticulously removed using a sharp needle. Foreign bodies involving the axial cornea should be removed with particular care to avoid scarring in this critical area. Antibiotic drops and cycloplegics should be instilled and a firm pad and bandage applied. Foreign bodies lodged deeply within the cornea require to be carefully removed under magnification occasionally with the assistance of a magnet under an operating microscope. Some foreign bodies projecting into the anterior chamber of the eye necessitate removal by an intra-ocular route under general anaesthesia.

Corneo-scleral lacerations

Non-perforating

Non-perforating corneal or scleral lacerations require no surgical treatment if they are superficial and the wound edge is well apposed. A firm pad and bandage usually provides sufficient external splintage for most corneal wounds. Deep corneal or scleral lacerations require careful suturing under an operating microscope using 8/0 Virgin silk for scleral lacerations and 10/0 monofilament nylon for corneal lacerations.

Perforating

Perforating injuries of the eye are ophthalmic emergencies and should be dealt with immediately by an experienced ophthalmologist. Wounds should be repaired accurately so as to restore normal shape and refractive properties of the globe. Perforating injuries of the eye take priority over lacerations of the eyelid and face and should be treated before any manipulation of facial fractures as external pressure may precipitate loss of intra-ocular content and irreparable damage to vision. Perforating corneal or scleral wounds may be associated with a retained intra-ocular foreign body and all such patients should have X-ray evaluation and localization of foreign bodies. Prolapsed and incarcerated uveal tissues, lens remnants or vitreous should be meticulously removed from the wounds and infection controlled with local and systemic antibiotics. Intra-ocular organization should be kept to a minimum by the judicious use of local and systemic corticosteroids. Posterior scleral perforations typically involve the retina and require special precedures to prevent subsequent retinal detachment, i.e. cryotherapy and techniques to reduce the volume of the posterior globe. Where a severe perforating injury has resulted in intra-ocular disorganization, inflammation and loss of vision enucleation may be advisable in view of continuing discomfort and the risk of sympathetic opthalmia. Between 15 per cent and 20 per cent of eyes with perforating wounds are eventually enucleated.

If a serviceable eye is retained long-term treatment will be directed towards preservation of clarity of the axial media and regaining normal refractive properties of the eye. Additional procedures may be needed to prevent retinal detachment and secondary glaucoma.

Intra-ocular foreign bodies

Most intra-ocular foreign bodies are metallic or glass and result from metal or stone being struck with a hammer or during the shattering of a windscreen during a road traffic accident. An intra-ocular foreign body should be suspected if there is a history of 'hammer and chisel injury', evidence of a small perforating corneal or scleral laceration, a localized iris tear or lens opacity or intra-ocular haemorrhage. With rare exception all intra-ocular foreign bodies should be removed as they may cause severe damage secondary to siderosis, infection or uveitis. Intra-ocular foreign bodies can be accurately localized either by direct examination or radiological and ultrasound techniques. Magnetic foreign bodies can be conveniently extracted using a hand or giant magnet, however, non-magnetic foreign bodies must be removed by direct means, e.g. intra-ocular forceps or by vitrectomy. These techniques are difficult, require hospitalization and may be complicated by cataract, retinal detachment, glaucoma and endophthalmitis.

Ocular contusions

Blunt injuries to the eyes are common and have particularly serious consequences for vision. They may cause intra-ocular haemorrhage, cataract, secondary glaucoma, retinal detachment and serious damage to the optic nerve.

Patients with significant hyphaemas (blood in the anterior chamber of the eye) require admission and observation. Secondary haemorrhage which occasionally occurs within two to five days is often associated with glaucoma and may require active therapy. Following resolution of intra-ocular haemorrhage full ocular examination is required to exclude glaucoma, cataract and peripheral retinal detachment. A vitreous haemorrhage following contusional injury to the eye should alert the physician to the likely pressure of an occult posterior scleral rupture or retinal tear or detachment. Admission, bedrest and observation is required. Scleral ruptures if present should be repaired and any retinal dehiscence identified and sealed. A retinal detachment if present will require immediate therapy and long-term follow up.

Injuries to the orbit

Perforating injuries

Perforating injuries of the orbit are uncommon but may be associated with damage to the eye and brain. If a projectile or perforating object has breached the bony orbit, neurological evaluation and radiology of the skull and orbit should be undertaken. Combined exploration of the orbit and cranial cavity may be required. If the bony orbit is intact and eye uninjured the wound should be explored, foreign bodies removed and necrotic tissue excised. Defects in the orbital fascia should be closed with 5/0 or 6/0 plain catgut and any extra-ocular muscle damage repaired. Foreign bodies with the exception of deeply embedded glass or plastic particles should be removed.

Fracture of the orbital margins

Most fractures of the orbital have no serious visual consequences unless the eye is damaged. Most fractures of the orbital wall, despite involving the paranasal sinuses, heal satisfactorily and without complication and merely require systemic antibiotic therapy to prevent secondary infections. Fractures of the orbital margin not associated with ocular disturbance or change in the patient's binocular status require repair only if cosmetically unacceptable.

Blow-out fractures of the orbit

Direct blows to the orbit may cause outward displacement of part of one of the bony walls of the orbit usually leaving the anterior rim of the orbit intact. The inferior orbital wall is commonly involved although occasionally the medial walls may be implicated. A blow-out fracture of the inferior orbital wall is characterized by orbital swelling and haemorrhage, surgical emphysema of the orbital and cheek tissus and infra-orbital paraesthesia or anaesthesia. The patient may experience diplopia in any position of gaze but particularly on looking down. Entrapment of the inferior orbital contents in the fracture may result in limitation of passive movement of the globe. Severe blow-out fractures may be associated with enophthalmus or exophthalmos and contusional injuries of the globe. X-rays of orbit with appropriate tomography will identify the nature and extent of the blow-out fractures. Systemic antibiotics should be prescribed and the patient observed. If there is persistent severe enophthalmus and diplopia surgical exploration and reconstruction of the inferior orbital wall may be necessary. Incarcerated tissue is mobilized and the defect closed using either a thin metallic or plastic plate fixed to the inferior orbital wall.

In the vast majority of blow-out fractures the orbital swelling resolves in a few weeks and ocular movements return to normal or near normal. If diplopia persists over a long period of time extra-ocular muscle surgery may be required to achieve a comfortable field of binocular single vision in the primary position.

Optic nerve injuries

Optic nerve injuries usually accompany head injuries with or without fractures of the upper face and skull. There is sudden loss of vision, ipsilateral dilatation of the pupil, and, after a few weeks, optic atrophy becomes apparent. X-ray generally confirms fractures of the middle third of the face and occasionally a bony abnormality of the optic canal. Surgical repair has generally been unrewarding and treatment should be restricted to the use of systemic corticosteroids and intravenous urea or Mannitol to reduce nerve oedema and relieve pressure on the intracanicular portion of the optic nerve.

Injuries of the lacrimal apparatus

The lacrimal gland is only rarely involved in injuries and no treatment is usually required, complications are rare. Injuries to the lacrimal canaliculae and sac are on the other hand common and require careful evaluation and repair. In general, as long as one canaliculus remains patent epiphora will be only marginal and repair of the second canaliculus should not implicate the intact canaliculus. A torn or ruptured canaliculus may be repaired by direct apposition of the severed ends, or if this is not possible the canaliculus is kept patent by leaving a nylon thread or silastic tube *in situ* for up to six months. Injuries to the lacrimal sac can be directly repaired and carry a good prognosis if the canaliculae are involved. Occasionally a dacryocystorhinostomy may be necessary if a distal obstruction of the lacrimal passages develops.

8 Ear, nose and throat

THE EAR

Outer ear

There are two dominant principles in the management of trauma to the pinna. First, the dangers of perichondritis following which the ear can be ugly and mis-shapen and secondly, the need to preserve as much skin and cartilage as possible because of the difficulties in correcting cosmetic deformities. Debridement, therefore, should be careful but not excessive, sutures should be through skin and not cartilage, and antibiotic cover should be provided if the wound has been contaminated.

Haematoma can lead to a cauliflower ear; evacuation, under strict aseptic procedure, is indicated, followed by a firm compression dressing. When lacerations involve a significant part of the skin of the external auditory meatus careful specialist attention is necessary to avoid the development of meatal stenosis.

Tympanic membrane

Rupture of the tympanic membrane can result from: (a) sudden changes of air pressure either from within the ear, via the Eustachian tube or from the external auditory meatus following a slap on the ear or an explosion; (b) water as in misdirected syringing or a mistimed dive; or (c) injury from a solid such as a hairpin.

The basic management is the same. Keep water out of the ear and leave it strictly alone unless there is contaminated debris, which should be removed by an ENT surgeon, or the ear is infected, when antibiotics should be prescribed. Ear drops are almost never indicated in traumatic rupture of the tympanic membrane.

Temporal bone fracture

There are two main types of fracture of the temporal bone, longitudinal and transverse. Radiology is not reliable in diagnosing these and the presence of blood in the middle ear behind an intact tympanic membrane or bleeding from the ear in the absence of an obvious external laceration, indicates a base of skull fracture, even in the absence of positive radiological findings. *Longitudinal* fracture, which is the more common, is usually associated with bleeding from the ear canal, a mild degree of conductive deafness, some high tone sensorineural deafness and, of course, any other signs relevant to such a head injury. There may, in addition, be leakage of CSF from the ear canal. Masterly inactivity is the secret of the management of the ear in these cases. Do not clean out the ear unless there is obvious contamination or infection. Do not prescribe antibiotics unless there is CSF, otorrhoea or obvious infection.

The tympanic membrane is usually intact in *transverse* fractures but blood is seen beyond it in the middle ear. The patient is extremely dizzy with nystagmus to the opposite side and with vomiting. There is severe sensorineural deafness and tinnitus. Assuming that there are no contra-indications, some form of labyrinthine sedative, e.g. cyclizine 50 mg IM, should be prescribed for the patient's comfort. The dizziness will eventually resolve but the deafness will be permanent.

The *facial nerve* is at risk in both these conditions and facial paralysis may be either immediate or delayed. The prognosis and management of these two types of facial paralysis are quite different and it is important to differentiate between them. Therefore facial nerve function must be assessed on admission. If there is immediate facial paralysis, surgical exploration of the nerve will be indicated when the patient's general condition permits. In delayed paralysis the prognosis is better and exploration is less likely to be required. Prompt referral to the ENT department is indicated.

The inner ear

There is no clear evidence that drugs alter the recovery of sensorineural deafness following trauma. However, in severe deafness following blast injury it is better to give the patient the benefit of any doubt that exists and immediate referral to the ENT department is indicated.

Barotrauma

Following descent in an aeroplane there may be severe pain in the ear due to the low middle ear pressure relative to atmospheric pressure. This is readily relieved by autoinflation by the Valsalva manoeuvre. If this fails the patient's pain and deafness can be relieved simply by puncturing the tympanic membrane with a hypodermic needle.

THE NOSE

Fracture of the nasal bones

Unless there is displacement or haematoma formation, nasal fractures do not require any specific treatment. Therefore, there is no indication for routine X-rays of the nasal bones in nasal trauma. Nasal fractures are easily manipulated within the first few hours but if there is delay beyond this time swelling develops and reduction should be further delayed for five to ten days. Beyond ten days it may be difficult to mobilize the nasal bones to get a satisfactory position.

Epistaxis

Epistaxis may be severe following trauma to the nose but usually settles spontaneously. If not, an anterior nasal pack should be inserted remembering that the floor of the nose is horizontal and that initial packing should be placed far back, building up in layers. If this fails to control the bleeding an ENT surgeon should be called.

Middle third fractures of the face

These are much more serious and may be associated with blood in the maxillary sinus, a blow-out fracture of the orbit or CSF rhinorrhoea. These require prompt specialist treatment and may involve the facial-maxillary surgeon, the ophthalmologist, the neurosurgeon or the otolaryngologist.

Haematoma of the septum

A septal haematoma, if left undrained, will lead, at best, to thickening of the septum and at worst to a septal abscess. These cases should be referred promptly to the otolaryngologist for drainage and continued care.

THE THROAT

Mouth and pharynx

Lacerations of the tongue, soft palate and posterior pharyngeal wall will be treated on their merits. Some of these are superficial and do not require any treatment. Others are deeper and require sutures. It may be necessary to suture the tongue to control bleeding.

The larynx

Many patients with laryngeal injuries are dead on arrival because of airway obstruction. Intubation is not necessarily the answer to these airway problems because it may be impossible to pass a tube through the injured larynx. One must always be prepared to carry out an emergency tracheostomy on these cases, but bear in mind that a laryngotomy, through the crico-thyroid membrane, or even a very wide bore needle straight into the trachea, may be life-saving.

Foreign bodies in the ears, nose and throat

These often require specialist attention and extreme care must be exercised if there is any risk to the airway. Foreign bodies in the ears or nose can often be easily removed following three basic principles:

1   The patient must be co-operative.
2   The lighting must be adequate.
3   The appropriate instrument must be used. This is usually a blunt hook which is passed beyond the foreign body and then gently withdrawn.

9 Around the shoulder

Trauma to the shoulder is common in all age groups except infancy and early childhood when infection should be suspected. Trauma to the shoulder can occur during delivery and result in brachial plexus injury, referred to as Erb's palsy, with loss of abduction at the shoulder and an internal rotational deformity of the arm. The appearance of the shoulder is altered by acromio-clavicular dislocation producing a characteristic bump. 'Squaring off' of the shoulder indicates dislocation unless proven otherwise by X-ray. If doubt exists, X-ray the other shoulder. Always check for neurovascular complications e.g. deltoid palsy due to circumflex humeral nerve damage or a brachial plexus injury before manipulative or surgical intervention.

Specific injuries

Fracture of clavicle (collar bone)

There is usually an obvious or palpable deformity of the subcutaneous bone. Manipulative reduction is seldom required. Brace both shoulders back with slings and maintain length for three weeks to reduce deformity, and tighten slings frequently. Despite this, a lump may occur but the cosmetic result will be worse with surgery and the complication rate much higher.

Dislocation of acromio-clavicular joint

Incomplete
Strain or subluxation of A–C joint. The deformity is small as coraco-clavicular ligaments remain intact. Treat in a sling and mobilise early.

Complete
Displacement is greater and the clavicle very mobile due to rupture of the coraco-clavicular ligaments.
If in doubt take X-rays with weighted arm. Treat with operative repair, though results can be disappointing.

Fracture of scapula

Treat in sling and mobilise as pain permits.

Dislocation of shoulder

Anterior

This is the usual type. The shoulder has a typical squared off appearance. Always X-ray prior to reduction to rule out associated fractures. If simple, reduce by manipulation. There are two well know methods:

1 Kochers — a sequenceof external rotation, abduction, then adduction and internal rotation whilst traction is maintained.

2 The Hippocratic — whereby the head is levered into the glenoid by traction on the arm and with a foot in the axilla.

A general anaesthetic is almost always required to relax muscle spasm, but if immediate, or in the elderly, a reduction can be obtained by sustained traction. Post-reduction management is very important. Immobilise for three to four weeks in the under forty year old as this may diminish the likelihood of recurrent dislocation. Mobilise the shoulder much earlier in the over 40s to prevent shoulder stiffness.

Posterior

This is rare and occurs occasionally in epilepsy. It can be easily missed on X-ray unless an axillary view is taken.

Recurrent dislocation

It requires operative repair following reduction.

Fracture of greater tuberosity of humerus

This is usually treated in a sling unless the displacement is great when open reduction and internal fixation should be seriously considered.

Fracture of surgical neck of humerus

This can usually be treated conservatively. Especially in children a considerable degree of displacement can be accepted. In adults, if displacement is extreme, open reduction is required where manipulation fails.

Rupture of rotator cuff

Rupture of the superior aspect where the supraspinatous tendon is attached can occur with trauma or can occur spontaneously in the older patient. Active abduction is not possible. The 'drop arm sign' is positive, i.e. when the arm is passively elevated and then released it falls limply to the side. A subacromial bursogram will confirm the diagnosis. Operative repair is difficult and surprisingly recovery can occur with time if treated conservatively.

Rupture of long head of biceps

This is an intracapsular lesion which produces a sagging, prominent biceps belly. Deformity persists, but if ignored, no true disability occurs.

10 Around the elbow

With the possible exception of the jaw there is no joint in which stiffness causes more disability than the elbow. The elbow is really three joints — radio-humeral, humero-ulnar and superior radio-ulnar. When flexed 90 degrees and viewed from behind the elbow presents three bony landmarks which form the points of an equilateral triangle: the medial and lateral epicondyles of the humerus and the olecranon process of the ulna. Displacement of one in relation to the others can be recognized by comparing with the 'triangle' of the opposite elbow.

Three important nerves pass close to the elbow — radial laterally: ulnar postero-medially and median anteriorly.

In elbow injury expect pain, swelling, deformity and restriction of movement. The carrying angle is approximately 170 degrees, i.e. with the elbow extended the forearm is normally in about 10 degrees of valgus. The normal flexion extension range is 0 degrees (straight) to 150 degrees (full flexion). The normal range of pronation and supination is 90 degrees each. As well as those features of the elbow itself, always check:

1 Distal circulation.

2 Nerve function: motor and sensory, radial, median and ulnar.

3 X-ray is always essential (when possible a true lateral at 90 degrees flexion and AP in as full extension as possible). If X-ray does not appear to show expected damage (especially in children) always *X-ray the opposite elbow in exactly the same projections and compare.*

Dislocation

1 Simple, posterior. Easily reduced under general anaesthetic; then Plaster of Paris back slab for about three weeks and then mobilisation by *active* movement only.

2 Accompanied by fracture (of capitellum, coronoid or head of radius) *may* require open reduction and/or internal fixation.

3 Dislocation of radial head alone (humero-ulnar joint undisturbed) may be congenital; or may imply a fracture of the shaft of the ulna (Monteggia injury) which may be missed if X-ray is not sufficiently distal.

Fractures

Lower end of humerus

(a) Adults — intercondylar and comminuted. Comminuted fractures in particular may best be treated conservatively, initially with a sling or collar and cuff, and later by active movement. Simple single fractures if displaced may require open reduction;

(b) Children — supracondylar. The commonest cause of Volkmann's ischaemic contracture — a catastrophic but usually avoidable complication. It results from impaired circulation in the anterior compartment of the forearm and can result in *permanent* nerve and muscle damage. The earliest sign is *pain*, this may be aggravated by passive extension of the fingers. Of the other classical 'p's', pallor and paralysis are late signs — perhaps too late, and pulseless, though a warning signal demanding careful observation is not by itself an indication for intervention. In supracondylar fracture a laterally displaced lower humeral fragment almost falls into place and is stable in a collar and cuff, but a medially displaced fragment may be very difficult to keep reduced. Plaster is not the answer but Dunlop traction is. Traction should also be used if flexion of the elbow causes impairment of the circulation. There is no place for plaster in the treatment of supracondylar fractures and probably rarely any indication for open operation except when signs of ischaemia persist even with the elbow extended, then here the brachial artery should be explored.

Summary of treatment

1 Check nerves and circulation before reduction.
2 General anaesthetic.
3 Reduce media or lateral displacement.
4 Flex elbow and apply collar and cuff.
(a) if this causes ischaemia abandon manipulation, apply skin traction with elbow sufficiently extended to restore hand circulation OR
(b) If the circulation remains satisfactory check X-ray *before discontinuing the anaesthetic*. If the position is not acceptable decide whether to carry out further manipulation under the same anaesthetic or switch to treatment by traction.

Head of radius

Fractures of the head or neck of radius often require surgery, open reduction, internal fixation or excision of fragments of the whole head. In young children displacement of the head of the radius due to fracture of the neck is easily missed due to the small ossific centre on the X-ray. X-ray the other elbow — always X-ray both elbows in children for comparison.

Olecranon

Fractures of the olecranon almost always require internal fixation.

Epiphyseal injuries

Injuries to the lower humeral epiphysis are always more extensive than X-ray sugggests and are sometimes missed altogether because the fragment may be almost entirely composed of cartilage. If in doubt X-ray opposite elbow. These injuries, unlike most fractures in children, often require open reduction and internal fixation to restore accurate articular surface and prevent non-union, growth disturbance and late deformity. The two fragments most commonly displaced are:
1 Capitellum plus half trochlea.
2 Medial epicondyle — sometimes trapped in joint, sometimes accompanied by ulnar nerve damage.

Tennis elbow

It is probably uncommon for this condition (lateral epicondylitis) or 'Golfer's Elbow' (medial epicondylitis) to result from a single acute injury.

Pulled elbow

It is reported that a sudden jerk of the elbow in a young child can result in the head of the radius slipping out of the articular ligament. It is further claimed that the displacement can be reduced simply by supinating the forearm. All other possible causes for the symptoms and signs in an injured child's elbow *must* be excluded before making this hypothetical and possiby dangerous diagnosis.

Summary

Check the circulation and the three nerves. In any case of doubt X-ray both elbows. Never use a complete plaster cast. In fact be very careful with bandages; as far as possible leave nothing across the flexor aspect of the elbow, e.g. a plaster of Paris back slab should be bandaged to the arm above the elbow and to the forearm below but not fixed with bandages around the elbow itself. A case of Volkmann's contracture has resulted from a plaster applied to 'treat' a 'fracture' of the olecranon which was nothing more than the normal epiphyseal line!

11 Around the wrist

The management of wrist injuries must be primarily directed towards preservation of hand function.

Soft tissue injuries

Penetrating injuries

Dorsal

Penetrating injuries of the back of the wrist are usually easier to fully diagnose and treat than volar surface injuries. The two main structures likely to be damaged are the veins and extensor tendons. Usually damage to the dorsal veins can be ignored. Evidence of extensor tendon damage to the fingers and thumb should be carefully sought by checking extensor action. Wrist extension (both ulnar and radial) should also be checked. Primary extensor tendon repair can often be performed using monofilament nylon or similar material. Postoperative splintage is required.

Volar

Diagnosis of this type of penetrating injury must be meticulous. It has two main components (a) careful inspection of the wound; if this is deep, a general anaesthetic will often be required, and (b) examination of hand and wrist function. The main structures likely to be damaged are arteries, flexor tendons and nerves.

Arterial damage. This occurs when either or both the radial and ulnar arteries may be cut. Repair should be carried out.

Flexor tendon damage. It requires examination of wrist flexion (both radial and ulnar) and of flexion at all joints in the fingers and thumb. It is often proper to proceed immediately to flexor tendon repair at the wrist.

Nerve damage. A careful examination of touch and pin prick sensation in the hand should be performed. If nerve damage is identified the nerve may be repaired primarily or later depending upon the skill of the surgeon. Following repair of arteries, tendons or nerves, immobilisation of wrist and hand is required in a position which will relieve the tension at suture lines in repaired structures.

Non-Penetrating injury

This is the very common 'sprained wrist'. X-ray will normally be required to exclude a fracture. Care must be taken to exclude a fractured scaphoid which may not be evident on the initial film. If there is marked tenderness in the anatomical snuff box even in the absence of a radiological fracture, a scaphoid type plaster of Paris should be applied. This is removed in 10–14 days and if the X-ray is still negative a fracture is unlikely to be present. However, if there is still tenderness in the anatomical snuff box apply a plaster for a further two weeks and re-X-ray. Normally, strapping with an elastic adhesive bandage for two to three weeks is adequate for a sprained wrist.

Fractures

X-ray are not a substitute for clinical examination in the diagnosis of wrist fractures. The correct X-rays can only be requested if a careful clinical assessment has taken place.

Colles' fracture

This is the classical injury of the elderly. It is a dorsiflexion injury usually caused by falling on the outstretched hand. There is a characteristic 'dinner-fork' deformity of the wrist. Immediate reduction under local or general anaesthetic is required. A short-arm plaster of Paris is applied from knuckles to just below the elbow. It is essential that the metacarpophalangeal joints should be able to flex to 90 degrees after application of the plaster of Paris. Postoperative elevation is sometimes needed for 24 hours. A check X-ray should be taken at one week and the plaster of Paris can usually be removed at five weeks.

Smith's fracture

Sometimes called a 'reverse Colles'', with volar displacement of the distal radius. This is a more unstable fracture and usually requires a long-arm plaster of Paris extending above the elbow.

Comminuted fracture

This is much more serious than a simple Colles' or Smith's fracture. The risk of wrist stiffness is greater after the fracture has healed.

Slipped lower radial epiphysis

This is the childhood equivalent of the Colles' fracture. Treatment is similar although splintage may be for as little as three weeks in the young child.

Fracture scaphoid

Already mentioned under 'sprained wrist'. A scaphoid plaster of Paris must include the thumb. Immobilisation may be needed for nine weeks. If the fracture is displaced it must be reduced preferably by closed methods and immobilised in a scaphoid plaster of Paris. If irreducible by closed manipulation it should be reduced by operation and fixed with a screw.

Fracture scaphoid — tubercle

This is really a ligamentous insertion injury and is not as serious as a wrist fracture. Strapping or a short period in plaster of Paris is usually adequate.

Carpal bone dislocation

Various dislocations of the carpal bones can occur with or without a scaphoid fracture. The trans-scaphoid perilunar fracture dislocation requires initially a closed reduction often followed by internal fixation of the scaphoid.

Rehabilitation after wrist injuries

There is no point in producing a perfectly healed fracture with permanently stiff fingers. Rehabilitation must begin at the latest, the day after injury. All splintage should be the minimum required to properly fulfill its purpose. All joints in the upper limb which are not immoblished must be exercised. The patient should be encouraged to begin using the hand for light everyday use as soon as post-traumatic oedema has begun to subside — after the first three to four days from injury. After removal of splintage, unless the patient has a rapid improvement in function in the first one to two weeks, physiotherapy may be required.

12 The hand

The location of a hand wound should alert the examiner to possible damage to important underlying structures.

Skin

Wounds may be closed by suture or by skin graft. Finger tip injury must be regarded with respect. Good healing is the aim of treatment. The finger tip wound should be closed primarily if possible. Bone must be trimmed back to avoid prominences in the finger pulp which would give a tender finger tip. If skin grafting is necessary then full thickness skin graft is recommended.

Blood vessels

A divided radial or ulnar artery at the wrist should be repaired as loss of one major vessel to the hand gives cold intolerance or exercise ischaemia. A digital artery should be repaired if possible if there is doubtful circulation to the digit.

Nerves

Nerve injury is diagnosed by testing motor and sensory function in the hand. Exploration of a wound is necessary if there is loss of nerve function. All divided nerves should be repaired primarily unless there are definite contraindications.

Tendons

Flexors

Loss of active finger flexion indicates injury to the flexor tendon. In the presence of a wound, exploration is indicated to establish the degree of injury. Division of the flexor tendon should be treated by primary repair. If both tendons are divided they should be repaired. Flexor tendon repair should be completed within forty-eight hours if possible. Closed tendon rupture should also be repaired as a primary procedure within forty-eight hours. Postoperatively the hand is splinted in flexion for three and a half weeks. After this the fingers are actively mobilized.

Extensors

Lacerations are repaired and splinted in extension for three and a half weeks. Extensor tendon rupture is usually treated by tendon transfer from adjacent tendons.

Bone and joint

The majority of hand fractures can be successfully treated considerably by plaster of Paris cast, Zimmer splint and neighbour strapping. However, fractures of the proximal and middle phalanges which are displaced may require open reduction and internal fixation. Intra-articular fractures, if they cannot be reduced by closed manipulation, require accurate open reduction, for example, the Bennett's fracture at the base of the first metacarpal. Internal fixation in the hand is by Kirschner wires in most cases. Plates and screws are only necessary in exceptional cases.

Collateral ligament instability requires splintage for three and a half weeks but the ulnar collateral ligament of the thumb often requires an operation. Volar plate injuries which are often indicated by small avulsion fractures at the base of the middle phalanx may lead to hyperextension and instability of the proximal interphalangeal joint unless splinted adequately. They should be splinted at 30 degrees of flexion at the proximal interphalangeal joint for three and a half weeks.

When splintage is applied to the whole hand the metacarpophalangeal joints should be flexed and the interphalangeal joints extended. The position of flexion of all joints must be avoided as this encourages stiffness.

Rehabilitation of the hand is all important. A stiff hand is virtually useless and all treatment must therefore be undertaken with a view to regaining full mobility. The preservation of one finger at the expense of loss of mobility of the hand as a whole is not justified. Rehabilitation must commence on the day following injury. If static splintage has been applied the patient must be assured of the necessity of his own efforts being all important in regaining function. Physiotherapy and occupational therapy is very helpful but cannot replace persistent repeated daily exercises by the patient. The patient must be left in no doubt that the end result depends on his or her own personal efforts.

13 Around the hip

Fractures of the upper end of the femur

These are common injuries, frequently seen in elderly patients and can be classified into three distinct types:
1 Intracapuslar.
2 Extracapsular (trochanteric).
3 Subtrochanteric.

Intracapsular fractures

These are frequently referred to as transcervical or subcapital in type (fractures at the base of the neck of the femur are technically partly intra-capsular). They are commonly found in the elderly patient frequently with concurrent osteoporosis and some authorities believe that the fracture may occur prior to the fall which is frequently given in history. Very occasionally these patients are able to walk following injury.

Diagnosis

Diagnosis is made clinically, first on the history and secondly on the appearance of the limb. The limb is usually held in external rotation with slight shortening and a minimum of bruising in the region of the hip. Diagnosis is confirmed by X-ray and at this stage the degree of displace-ment of the fracture can be estimated. Garden classified these from Stage 1 to Stage 4 depending on the degree of displacement; Stage 4 being totally displaced and unlikely to have any soft tissue bridge across the fracture. It is advisable at the stage of X-raying these patients to have a routine chest X-ray performed as there are frequently concurrent medical problems.

Management

Management is based initially on first-aid, gentle longitudinal traction to the limb relieving pain and permitting movement. But in general terms all of these fractures should be treated surgically.

Undisplaced fractures. The *undisplaced* fractures (Garden 1 or 2) are best managed by any form of internal fixation, the traditional Smith–Peterson pin, may still be used though there is a trend away from this towards devices that are screwed into the neck of the femur (Garden or Richards).

Displaced fractures. For *displaced* fractures (Garden 3 or 4) the physical state of the patient will often determine the surgical management. In a very decrepit, elderly person simple femoral head replacement may be the best management (Austin Moore or Thompson) though this prosthesis does not function well in an active patient. In younger patients who are more active, closed reduction in the operating theatre followed by internal fixation of some means (generally a screw of some type) is the treatment of choice. Internal fixation should not be performed unless a satisfactory reduction is achieved. Occasionally open reduction of the fracture is required. Some authorities believe that for the active, elderly patient a total hip replacement is the best and surest method of achieving satisfactory mobilisation of the patient. The object of management is to have the patient up and walking as soon as possible and this should be possible within three or four days from the surgery.

These fractures are occasionally encountered in younger patients and rarely in children. Any patient under the age of fifty suffering from an intracapsular fracture should be regarded as an absolute emergency and surgical treatment should be instituted immediately.

Complications

1 General — Pressure sores, pneumonia, retention of urine, renal failure, deep venous thrombosis, pulmonary embolism.
2 Delayed and non-union — these are rare nowadays with better forms of internal fixation but are still a recognised complication of displaced fractures.
3 A vascular necrosis is seen particularly following displaced fractures and this leads to osteoarthritis.

Extracapsular fracture (trochanter)

These fractures frequently occur with a heavy fall on to the region of the greater trochanter and are frequently found in the elderly. In general, the quality of the bone is better than in those patients with intracapsular fractures.

Usually the patient is unable to walk and the limb is held in an externally rotated position, though shortening can be more marked in these cases than in intracapsular fractures and on palpation of the hip region there is often palpable thickening of the greater trochanter. The principles of management of these patients is the same as with intracapsular fractures and virtually all of these patients require operative treatment. Usually a blade plate is inserted to stabilize the fracture. Occasionally these fractures are unstable (particularly when the lesser trochanter is involved in the fracture) and more complex forms of fixation can be required. Rehabilitation is as with intracapsular fractures.

Complications

1 Delayed and non-union are extremely rare.
2 Malunion is extremely common where inadequate or no internal fixation is used. The neck shaft angle is reduced and coxa vara is the result. Occasionally this can occur secondary to failure of the implant to hold the fracture.
3 A vascular necrosis rarely occurs.

Sub-trochanteric fractures

These are much less common than the above two types of fracture and they are occasionally seen secondary to a metastatic deposit in this region. These can be very difficult fractures to manage because the proximal fragment of the femur is flexed and abducted by muscle pull. Generally operative treatment is advised, either a blade plate or some form of intramedullary nail.

The complications of this fracture are either failure of the fixation device to hold the fracture adequately or, if the failure is treated by conservative means, it may result in malunion.

Less usual fractures of the upper femur

Fractures of the greater trochanter do occur, seen frequently in the elderly and of little significance, the patient requiring rest until the pain settles and then mobilisation. Fractures of the lesser trochanter are occasionally encountered as isolated injuries. Great intention should be paid to these patients as there may be underlying pathology such as a metastatic deposit.

Traumatic dislocations of the hip joint

These are not uncommon injuries and are of three main types:
1 Posterior.
2 Anterior.
3 Central.
There are other rare dislocations of the hip such as obturator and scrotal.

Posterior dislocation of the hip

These injuries are frequently associated with fractures of the pelvis and particularly of the posterior lip of the acetabulum. They are not uncommon injuries and typically seen in road accidents where the driver or front seat passenger of a car strikes the dash board with his knee with the hip flexed at 90 degrees forcing the hip to dislocate posteriorly. The degree of injury to the posterior lip of the acetabulum depends on the degree of flexion of the hip at the time of the injury.

Diagnosis

Diagnosis is made in these patients clinically by the appearance of the limb. It is usually slightly flexed, internally rotated and short. There may be concurrent injury to the knee joint.

A common complication initially in these patients is damage to the sciatic nerve, particularly where a fracture is present. Diagnosis of the dislocation is confirmed by X-ray. The size of the lesser trochanter will indicate in which direction rotation has occurred (if it has disappeared there is internal rotation, if it is more prominent there is external rotation). Internal rotation in conjunction with dislocation on X-ray indicates a posterior dislocation. Further X-rays including oblique views of the pelvis, as well as a lateral view may be required but these patients are frequently in severe pain.

Management

Management is based on early closed reduction of the patient with a pure dislocation without fracture and without sciatic nerve involvement. If there is a severely fractured acetabulum in association and the sciatic nerve is not functioning there is a very strong case for early open reduction to avoid further damage to the nerve. The knee joint should be examined under anaesthesia for damage to ligaments, particularly the posterior cruciate ligament, and following reduction of the hip joint, a gentle assessment of its stability should be made.

Postoperative management by tradition entailed six weeks skin traction with bedrest to allow healing of soft tissues. Where there is no fracture present some patients may be immobilised earlier. Where there is gross damage to the posterior acetabular lip, operative repair with screws may be required.

Complications

Complications following posterior dislocation or fracture dislocations are not uncommon, vascular necrosis of the head of the femur and osteoarthritis being the two most important. Osteoarthritis is likely to occur where there is an associated fracture. A vascular necrosis is particularly likely to occur where the severity of injury is greater, and especially if the head or neck of femur is fractured in association with this dislocation. Delay in achieving reduction may predispose the patient to a higher risk of developing a vascular necrosis.

Anterior dislocation

This is a much rarer dislocation and was typically seen in coal miners suffering a hyperextension injury of the hip. Fractures are much less common with these patients and close reduction can be extremely difficult. Typically the limb is short and externally rotated, though the degree of shortening is less than with posterior dislocation. The same principles of management apply and the same complications though the lower rate of fracture in association with these injuries makes the incidents of osteoarthritis less.

Central dislocation

These are seen typically following a very heavy fall on to the trochanteric region. The force of the injury drives the head of femur into the pelvis. These can be associated with more serious pelvic fractures. Clinically there may be little to find in these patients apart from swelling and bruising over the greater trochanter. There will be loss of movement in the hip joint, slight shortening in severely displaced cases but generally no rotational abnormality. X-rays will confirm the diagnosis. Frequently oblique pelvic views will be required to verify the extent of the pelvic fracture.

Management

Management can be extremely difficult but basically traction should be applied to try to reduce the hip joint and allow fibrocartilage to fill the medial defect. The outlook for many of these hips is for osteoarthritis to develop and subsequent operative management of this complication is made easier if the hip joint is kept concentrically reduced. Occasionally traction with a metal pin through the greater trochanter can aid this though generally longitudinal traction (either skin or skeletal) is satisfactory.

Epiphyseal injuries

Any of the epiphyses around the hip can be injured:
1 The upper femoral epiphysis.
2 The greater trochanter.
3 The lesser trochanter.
4 The ischial tuberosity.
5 The anterior iliac spine.

The upper femoral epiphysis

Slipped under femoral epiphysis (SUFE) is rarely traumatic in origin. It is a condition typically seen between the ages of ten–fifteen, slightly more common in boys, and in girls never seen after the onset of menstruation. The patients are frequently fat or tall or have signs of endocrine abnormality (Frolich) and in general present either acutely, chronically or as an acute-on-chronic situation. Many present with pain in the knee. Occasionally when seen outside the normal age spectrum for this condition one should suspect pituitary abnormalities.

Typically the epiphysis displaces posteriorly relative to the neck of the femur and this results in an external rotation abnormality of the hip joint and on attempting to flex the hip the external rotation abnormality becomes more marked. X-rays should be taken in two planes, the lateral view being the most important.

One should always be aware that the contralateral hip can undergo the same pathology even when the patient is resting in bed.

Management

Management of this condition is based on prevention of further deformity. Reduction should not be attempted, pins are passed along the neck of the femur into the epiphysis under X-ray control and if there is gross endocrine abnormality in the patient the contralateral hip should be pinned prophylactically. The patient is usually mobilised on the crutches as soon as the wound has healed and the pins are left *in situ* until the epiphyseal line closes on radiological examination. Where major deformity persists in the upper end of the femur these pins should still be inserted to avoid further slip and corrective osteotomy lower in the femur in the region of the trochanters should be performed later. Only in the rare acute traumatic case should manipulative reduction be attempted.

Complications

1 A vascular necrosis of the capital epiphysis is never seen in untreated cases and must be considered an iatrogenic phenomenon probably secondary to manipulation.
2 Chondrolysis can occur for no apparent reason and is shown clinically be persistence of pain in the region of the hip and on X-ray examination by loss of the cartilage space in the joint. The joint remains extremely stiff for some years but many of these patients appear to be able to reform their cartilage space on X-ray at least to a satisfactory extent, though they may need to use crutches for two years or more.
3 Osteoarthritis cases which are severely displaced are left with an incongruous upper end of femur and may require operative management in later life.

The greater trochanter

Avulsion of the greater trochanter is rare.

The lesser trochanter

Avulsion of this epiphysis is rare. Fractures of the lesser trochanter have been mentioned already.

The ischial-tuberosity

Avulsion of the ischial-tuberosity is seen in athletic adolescents; the hamstring muscles being the cause of the injury. Usually rest until pain settles is all that is required in these patients.

The anterior iliac spine

Avulsion of the anterior iliac spine (the origin of the straight head of rectus femoris) is occasionally encountered in young athletes. It may show on X-ray in later years as a spur of bone anterior to the hip joint.

14 The knee

Extensor mechanism

Injury may result from direct violence or sudden stresses.

1 Sprain of the tibial tubercle is also called Osgood–Schlatter's disease. It affects children aged eleven–fourteen years. Treatment is restriction of activities and in resistant cases a cylinder cast for about four weeks. Only rarely is surgery necessary.

2 Patellar tendon rupture results in an inability to extend the knee. There is a palpable defect below the patella and the patella is displaced somewhat superiorly. Surgical repair is necessary.

3 Fractured patella: (a) very comminuted, should be excised and the defect repaired; (b) a displaced transverse fracture may be repaired and fixed internally, usually by wire; (c) occasionally either the superior or inferior pole is excised and the remaining pole is sutured with wire to the adjacent soft tissues.

4 Quadriceps rupture is unusual. Surgical repair is indicated if the defect is large.

5 Acute dislocation of patella is diagnosed when an X-ray reveals an osteochondral fracture of lateral femoral condyle. The patella is reduced by extending the knee. The knee should be immobilised for several weeks. If the dislocation becomes recurrent surgical repair may become necessary. If a loose fragment of bone is noted it should be excised.

Ligaments

If ligament rupture is suspected the knee should be carefully assessed. The collateral ligaments are tested by flexing the knee to about twenty degrees and applying a valgus or varus strain. Stress X-rays under anaesthesia may be helpful. A positive anterior draw sign indicates rupture of the anterior cruciate ligament and/or the medial collateral ligament. A positive draw sign indicates rupture of the posterior cruciate ligament. Acute major ligament ruptures should be repaired surgically as far as possible. Chronic ligamentous laxity may be treated by tendon transposition and more recently by synthetic tendon replacement.

Menisci

These fibrocartilaginous structures spread the weight-bearing area between the femur and tibia. If they are torn and cause locking of the knee they should be excised. Diagnosis of a torn meniscus can be made by taking a careful history and carrying out a careful examination. Plain X-rays are necessary to rule out other causes of locking. Arthrography may be helpful and arthroscopy is becoming more popular.

Fractures

Supracondylar fractures of the femur, if displaced, may require open reduction and internal fixation. If 'T' shaped, accurate reduction of the condyles is necessary. Fractures of the tibial condyles, if displaced in young patients, should be treated by open reduction and internal fixation. In elderly patients a more conservative approach is usually taken and the fracture is treated by skeletal traction, early movement and late weight-bearing.

15 The ankle

In ankle injuries it is important to take an accurate history, carry out an examination and X-ray the ankle. Record any neurological or vascular deficit. It is important to remember that ankle injuries swell and if a plaster cast has to be applied, suitable precautions, such as elevation of the limb and splitting of the cast may have to be undertaken.

Soft tissues injuries

Ligamentous damage

The lateral ligament of the ankle is most commonly injured. This history, local swelling, tenderness and feeling of instability all point to rupture. If in doubt, stress X-rays of the ankle should be taken. Treatment may be by plaster cast or operative repair.

Ruptured Achilles tendon

Rupture of tendo Achilles is often missed. A sportsman often feels that he has been kicked from behind or someone running for a bus suffers a searing pain in the lower portions of the calf. On examination there is considerable disability with pain and local tenderness above the heel. There is weakness of plantar flexion of the ankle. Swelling is noted around the heel cord. A tendon defeat may be noted in the Achilles tendon. The patient if examined in the prone position may present a positive 'Squeeze Test'. Upon squeezing the normal calf with one hand the ankle is seen to plantar flex. When carried out on a calf with a ruptured Achilles tendon, plantar flexion does not occur. Treatment of the ruptured Achilles tendon is usually by direct surgical repair. Postoperatively a plaster cast is applied with the ankle in some degree of equinus for about two months. Plaster cast treatment alone is advocated by some authorities.

Bony injuries

Although these injuries are more dramatic especially when seen on X-rays, the possibility of other soft tissue injuries being present must be kept in mind. The simplest classification from a practical point of view is that of 'Stable fractures' and 'Unstable fractures'. The treatment of a stable fracture which is undisplaced and therefore does not require reduction is by a simple short-leg walking plaster cast for several weeks.

An unstable fracture may be associated with gross deformity, dislocation, neurovascular impairment, pressure on overlying skin and an open wound.

Treatment

1 Gross deformity is corrected by gentle manipulation and traction. This will reduce the pressure from the skin, the blood vessels and the nerves.

2 Dislocations should be reduced immediately.

3 Consideration is given to open reduction and internal fixation. Ligamentous repair may have to be combined with bony repair.

4 Open injuries should be treated by debridement. Depending on the state of the tissues internal fixation may be carried out early or later.

16 The foot

Any discussion of fracture dislocations should be based on a planned approach (e.g. the mode of injury, the management and complications, form a simple plan for both the student and practitioner). This approach should be considered when any fracture arrives at the receiving room door. In considering the mode of injury it is interesting to note that the foot is an excellent example of injuries caused by both direct and indirect violence. There is the comminuted os calcis fracture resulting from the fall from a height and the hallux fracture from a crushing injury as examples of direct violence, and again the severe injuries to the hind foot region involving the talus and adjacent joints is an excellent example of indirect violence. For convenience the foot injuries can be divided into three sites:

1 The forefoot including the toes and metatarsals.
2 The midfoot including the tarso-metatarsal joints, the navicular, cuboid and cuneiform bones.
3 The hindfoot including the talus, the surrounding joints and the os calcis.

Forefoot

Fractures of the phalanges of the outer four toes are common, they are often difficult to reduce; however an effort should be made with closed reduction, both with respect to fractures of the phalanges and inter-phalangeal or metatarso-phalangeal joint dislocations. The commonest fracture in this region as result of direct violence is the comminuted fracture of the distal phalanx of the hallux, the management of which is simple, with immobilization in a simple splint and attention to the often seen soft tissue damage. *Metatarsal fractures* are common, they can occur as a result of indirect violence, e.g. the March fracture. As a rule they are simply treated with strapping and protected weight bearing. On occasions grossly displaced fractures require an open reduction. This is particularly seen in multiple fractures of the metatarsal necks when transfixion with Kirschner wires can be useful and obviates the later complication of malunion and the necessity for metatarsal head excision at a later date. The common injury at this site is the so-called Dancer's fracture at the attachment of the *peroneus brevis* to the outer side of the base of the 5th metatarsal bone, another example of an indirect violence injury due to inversion. This fracture is simply managed by either strapping or in painful cases a below-knee plaster immobilization. It can be notoriously troublesome and occasionally proceeds to non-union. The long-term outlook is satisfactory and of course it should not be confused with the epiphyseal line in children.

Midfoot

Dislocation of the tarsometatarsal joints due to either direct or indirect violence is not infrequently seen and unfortunately can be missed. It is obvious on clinical examination and simple manipulative reduction shortly after the injury is sufficient. Fractures of the cuneiform and cuboid bones are uncommon and are easily managed. Careful scrutiny of injuries to this region should be made to ascertain there is no question of any adjacent joint dislocation. This is particularly so in fractures of the navicular bone and in this fracture open reduction and internal fixation can be required for transverse fractures of the body. The commonest injury of this bone is a fracture of the tuberosity at the attachment of the tibialis posterior. This is a simple injury and requires little treatment.

Hindfoot

This is a very confusing subject and made more difficult by the numerous classifications described by various authors. A simple classification easily remembered is (a) dislocation of the talus on its own, (b) peritalar dislocations, (c) fractures of the talus with or without dislocation, (d) fractures of the os calcis.

Dislocation of the talus

This is due to indirect violence and can be produced by violent inversion of the foot, it is easily recognized on X-rays examination and is difficult to reduce. It is not infrequently compound. Open reduction is frequently required. Great care should be taken to preserve the talus and replace it in the ankle mortis as although avascular necrosis is a frequent complication at this site revascularization is often seen and has been recorded on several occasions.

Peritalar dislocations

For simplicity these can occur at the subtaloid joint or the talo-navicular joint. They are as a result of an inversion injury of the foot and forefoot, the talus remaining intact in the ankle mortis and the dislocation occurring at either the subtaloid joint or at the talo-navicular joint. Manipulative reduction is as a rule straightforward, occasional examples of trapping of the adjacent tendons in the dislocated joint can obviate this and open reduction is on these occasions required. This should be carried out promptly as in the later described cases to avoid skin necrosis and vascular complications.

Fractures of the talus with or without dislocation

These are due to acute dorsiflexion of the foot at the ankle joint (better termed acute extension). The degree of injury is directly proportional to the violence incurred; at one end of the scale a simple fracture of the neck of the talus occurs without displacement due to impingement of the neck of the talus on the anterior articular margin of the lower end of the tibia; at the other end of the scale the injury results in separation of the talar fragments, dislocation of the subtaloid joint and a rotational injury to the talus so that the fracture surface of the body points towards the skin surface. Between the extremes of the scale a combination of these injuries can occur. Manipulative reduction is often difficult, it should be attempted with the ankle held in marked plantar flexion. Open reduction again is often required to re-establish the congruity and should be treated as an emergency.

Injuries to the os calcis

This is the classical example of a fracture due to indirect violence, the patient almost invariably giving a history of falling from a height on to a hard wooden or concrete surface. The fractures can be classified simply into those involvng the body as a whole including the tuberosity, and upper surface, and those involving the subtaloid joint. The latter can vary from simple fractures of the sustentaculum tali with slight to moderate displacement to comminuted fractures of the body as a whole, grossly involving the subtaloid and even the calcaneo-cuboid joints. Numerous methods of management have been described, including open reduction and primary arthrodesis of the joint through to totally conservative treatment. In severe cases the patient should be admitted to hospital, the affected limb or limbs should be elevated on a suitable board, if necessary for several days until the swelling subsides. When the subtaloid joint is not involved plaster immobilization is a simple and helpful method in the rehabilitation of the patient. Involvement of the subtaloid joint is as a rule better treated by protected weight bearing and graduated exercises from an early stage. Gross displacement with broadening of the heel can be managed by manipulation in the early stages, if only to facilitate shoe fitting. The injury is most often seen associated with industrial accidents and, curiously enough, later treatment in the form of triple fusion is not often required. *Remember to check for associated spinal injury.*

17 Shafts of long bones

The healing of fractures in the shafts of long bones of the body, which are of predominantly dense cortical bone, is fundamentally different from the healing of cancellous bone.

Fracture shaft of humerus

The mechanism of this injury is either a direct blow to the arm which causes associated soft tissue injury or an indirect force applied from a fall on the outstretched hand or elbow. In both cases a common complication is damage to the musculo-spiral nerve and a resultant wrist drop. Manipulative reduction of this fracture is seldom required. If the wrist is supported in a collar and cuff with the elbow in slightly more than 90 degrees of flexion, then an X-ray taken in this unsupported position will, in many cases, show a fracture in good alignment. Thus the action of gravity reduces the fracture and helps maintain it. The pull of gravity may be supplemented by a U-shaped plaster slab applied to the upper arm which also splints the fracture bone. The fracture usually heals in four to six weeks and only on rare occasions would excessive traction or interposition of soft tissues lead to non-union. During the time of immobilization, exercises of the fingers, wrist and pendulum and exercises for the shoulder are essential. If there has been damage to the muscular spiral nerve it should be treated expectantly (as a neuropraxia) and a lively splint applied. If the fracture results in non-union, early operative reduction, internal fixation with a plate and screws or intramedullary nailing is indicated, as an adjunct to the bone grafting procedure. Incipient or frank pathological fractures due to malignant disease respond well to internal fixation with intramedullary nails.

Fracture of the radial and ulnar shafts

The mechanism of this fracture is usually due to a direct blow on the arm which causes transverse fractures at a similar level, or indirect twisting forces in which case the fractures are usually at different levels in the parallel bones. In all cases the joints of the wrist and elbow must be clearly seen on X-ray. In children's fractures because of the nature of the bone, the fracture is usually of a greenstick type. Reduction under general anaesthetic is usually necessary and the arm is held in a long-arm plaster of Paris with three-point fixation, the wrist being pronated for a fracture of the lower third, neutral for a fracture of the middle third, and supinated for a fracture of the upper third. The fracture heals in three to five weeks, at which time the plaster may be removed.

In adult fractures over the age of fourteen the treatment is different. Because a good reduction is essential for function and is hard to hold by external methods, open reduction and internal fixation is usually carried out in all cases. Internal fixation is usually achieved by a plate and screws but may on occasion be held by intramedullary rods. Rigid internal fixation allows early mobilization and early return to full function. It may take up to twelve weeks for these fractures to heal in the adult.

In all cases of forearm fractures beware of the pale, paraesthetic, pulseless and increasingly painful hand. These signs indicate a compartmental syndrome which is a surgical emergency and failure to act may result in Volkmann's ischaemic contracture. Fracture of one of the bones of the forearm is unusual and X-ray should always be sought of the wrist and elbow joint to exclude a dislocated head of radius accompanying an isolated fracture of the ulna (Monteggia fracture) or dislocation of the distal ulna in association with an isolated fractured radius (Galeazzi fracture). In these types of fracture internal fixation by a plate and screw is indicated.

Fractured shaft of femur

The mechanism of this injury by a direct blow results in a transverse fracture with soft tissue injury, whereas indirect forces cause spiral fractures. Always beware of the pathological fracture in the older patient and in all cases of fractured femur the hips should be X-rayed to exclude a posterior dislocation; and in all cases of fractured femur the sciatic nerve function should be tested. Reduction of the fractured shaft of femur is usually achieved by traction and in an emergency skin traction in a Thomas' splint is satisfactory. Different methods of treatment may then be debated at leisure depending on various factors. Many cases can be managed over the period of healing of the fracture in a Thomas' splint, in a child using skin traction, in the adult using skeletal traction. In these cases it is essential to measure the leg daily for the initial period of treatment to ensure length and alignment.

In fractures of the upper third of the femur the proximal fragment is usually pulled into abduction, flexion and external rotation and these are usually managed in skeletal traction of the modified Hamilton-Russell type. In lower third fractures there is usually backward tilt of the distal fragment and these are managed in a Thomas' splint with skeletal traction, a knee flexion iron and posterior padding. In a number of circumstances internal fixation may be indicated.

In all cases, after the initial treatment, the fracture may be managed in a femoral cast brace and this method allows early mobilization of soft parts and ambulation of the patient, yet protecting the fractured bone while it heals. Healing in children usually takes six weeks, in the adult over twelve weeks.

Fractured tibia and fibula

The mechanism of injury may be direct causing a transverse fracture, or a twisting force applied to the foot causing a spiral fracture of tibia and fibula. Compound fractures are common due to the subcutaneous situation of the tibia. The fractures should be reduced under general anaesthetic and held in a long-leg plaster of Paris and the patient admitted for elevation of the limb.

At this time various methods of treatment can be discussed. If a good reduction has been achieved the treatment may be continued in a long-leg cast, followed in a few weeks by a walking heel to allow early weight-bearing. The long-leg cast may be changed for a patella tendon-bearing cast which would allow knee mobilization and ambulation. Unstable fractures may be treated in bed on a Bohler–Braun frame with skeletal traction through an os calcis pin followed by ambulation in a long-leg cast. In some cases internal fixation of these fractures is indicated usually by interfragmented screws or onlay plates. However, the incidence of infection in internal fixation in tibial fractures is unacceptably high. In severely traumatized limbs where there is skin and tissue loss or bone loss, an external fixateur may be used. Healing of the fractured tibia, especially in its lower third is very slow and one must always aim for a good reduction, adequate immobilization and early ambulation while the fracture heals. Isolated fibular fractures are usually associated with injuries of the ankle or knee and should be treated as such. Occasionally a direct blow to the fibula may result in an isolated fracture of the fibula, in which case a crepe bandage is sufficient for symptomatic relief while the fracture heals.

Section 3

18 Vascular injuries

In the past penetrating vascular injuries were usually a feature of military conflict. In recent times they have been increasingly noted in urban civilian populations and result from acts of violence, ranging from a solitary shooting or stabbing incident to injuries inflicted on a large scale by guerillas or militia using advance weaponry and explosive devices. Significant advances in the treatment of vascular injuries, as in other surgical fields, were made in wartime and newly–learned concepts extended to civilian practice.

In general, the civilian vascular surgeon has to deal with blunt or penetrating injuries to vessels occurring mainly as a consequence of road traffic, industrial or domestic accidents, and sometimes following invasive procedures in hospital. While military injuries occur almost exclusively in young males, civilian trauma may affect any age group, and treatment of vascular injury in the arteriosclerotic patient can be challenging. Vascular injury following blunt trauma is frequently accompanied by injuries to bone, vital organs and viscera. These blunt injuries to blood vessels and long bones, especially of the lower limbs, are often more difficult to manage than penetrating injuries.

The principles of management remain the same for battle casualties rushed to field hospitals or for patients admitted to a modern well-equipped and fully staffed metropolitan hospital. A major vessel injury endangers life and puts at risk the viability of tissues which it normally supplies. Therefore speed in diagnosis and operation is essential; rapid examination proceeding in concert with emergency treatment. The objectives of treatment are control of bleeding, resuscitation, wound toilet, restoration of circulation and prevention of complications. Operative treatment must ideally be undertaken by surgeons experienced in vascular reconstruction.

Mechanisms of injury

Penetrating

Penetrating injuries are caused by sharp objects such as knives and splinters of glass, by bullets of low or high velocity, or by fragments from explosive devices.

A high velocity missile (in excess of 762 m/sec or 2500 ft/sec) may penetrate the arterial wall sharply without stretching it, but even if it does not do so the temporary cavitational effect crushes, stretches and tears vessels which may or may not be directly in the path of the missile, in addition to sucking in fragments of dirt, clothing, skin and organism. A low velocity missile (under 304 m/sec or 1000 ft/sec) usually only disrupts and deforms a vessel in its path. It may therefore help to know the type of missile responsible. A shotgun discharged at close range will produce severe and extensive destruction of all tissues with much contamination. Various types of bombs and secondary missiles may cause extensive damage to blood vessels and surrounding tissues. In contrast, a stabbing may sever major vessels with minimal soft tissue injury.

Over the last decade, iatrogenic trauma to femoral, brachial and radial arteries has resulted from the wide use of needles and catheters for angiography, cardiac catheterization, arterial pressure monitoring, arterial blood sampling and percutaneous transluminal balloon angioplasty. The subclavian and carotid arteries may be injured during insertion of central venous catheters, brachial or stellate blocks or during surgery to correct the thoracic outlet syndrome. Orthopaedic procedures such as the removal of a herniated lumbar disc may occasionally produce catastrophic bleeding from the aorta and cava and their ramifications. Surgery to the hip, knees and shoulder joints may accidentally cause arterial injury through the use of a scalpel, drill or screws.

Blunt

With regard to blunt trauma, road traffic accidents account for the majority of vascular injuries. While direct vessel injury may sometimes occur, in most cases vascular damage results from fractures of long bones. The vulnerability of these vessels to powerful shear forces is greatest either at segments which lie next to a long bone or at points of relative fixity, especially in close proximity to joints. Bony fragments may lacerate a vessel or angulation at a fracture may stretch an artery, but the avulsive forces producing fracture dislocations, particularly at the knee, are notorius for serious traction injuries of adjacent vessels and nerves.

Crush

The crush syndrome, first recognized in wartime, usually followed the massive destruction by the weight of falling masonry after air-raids and bomb explosions. In peacetime, this clinical picture may be seen in industrial, mining and road traffic accidents. Crushed limbs, a crushed chest or abdomen may be associated with vascular injuries which are potentially fatal and represent a great challenge.

Chemical

Rarely, misplacement of a needle in the arm may result in the inadvertent intra-arterial injection of drugs such as thiopentone or diazepam. These agents will destroy the endothelium of the vessel, producing thrombosis, often with irreversible ischaemia; gangrene and eventual amputation. Drug addicts may inject a variety of chemical and pharmacological substances with resultant infection and gangrene of the hand and forearm.

Types of injury

Immediate

1 *Thrombosis in continuity* may follow a simple blunt injury or if the vessel lay close to the path of a high velocity bullet. Minimal endothelial damage or a small intimal tear is enough to provoke platelet and fibrin aggregation. In arteriosclerotic artery, conditions of reduced flow and patency will favour this outcome. The process is gradual and ischaemic changes may be slow to appear.

2 *Intimal flap* may occur following blunt injury to an unopened artery or after needling and catheterization procedures. The formation of an intimal flap may develop into a dissection with intramural bleeding which could go on to occlusion of the lumen.

3 *Intramural haematoma* may occasionally follow blunt injury although the vessel coats are intact. The size of the haematoma may be sufficient to occlude the artery.

4 *Spasm* is caused by contraction of the muscle wall; if segmental, it is usually associated with localised disruption of the endothelium or intima, but, if diffuse, it may be a feature of general vasoconstriction following haemorrhage.

5 *Traction* produces vessel elongation, intimal tears and separation from the media with resultant intramural bleeding and thrombosis. With progressive stretching, the media is disrupted and finally the remaining layer of adventitia may be pulled apart and, in doing so, retracts, plugging the ends of the vessels with relatively effective haemostasis. Distal ischaemia can be severe and pulses are usually not palpable.

6 *Laceration*, depending on the cause, may be a ragged or clean incisive tear in the wall through which blood is lost externally or into the surrounding tissues producing a haematoma. Spasm and intramural bleeding may be present locally but distal flow and pulses may be maintained.

7 *Defect in the wall* is really a partially severed artery with ragged edges and is so often caused by a high-velocity bullet or bomb fragment. As continuity of part of the arterial wall is maintained, circumferential contraction cannot take place. Consequently, bleeding may be rapidly exsanguinating or contained within a tense and even pulsatile haematoma through which recurrent bleeding may occur.

8 *Transection* or sharp division of a vessel by a cutting edge or gross disruption with a high-velocity missile will result in two severed ends. Here the circular muscles constrict and retract into adjoining tissue and a plug of thrombus is formed which propagates down the distal artery where collateral flow is very poor. Flow is interrupted and pulses cannot be felt.

Late

1 *False aneurysm* may follow laceration or damage to part of the arterial wall. Haemorrhage occurring within fascial confines forms a haematoma which undergoes organization and into which blood gradually forces its way to form a cavity lined by endothelium. This cavity circumscribed by fibrous tissue slowly expands but remains in continuity with the arterial lumen. Turbulent flow within this false aneurysm facilitates clot formation. The enlarging aneurysm may first obstruct adjacent veins or it may rupture. A thrill, systolic bruit and an obviously pulsatile mass, which is warm and may be tender in its early stages, are noted on examination.

2 *Arteriovenous fistula* is the communication established between an adjoining artery and vein which are injured simultaneously. Initially, arterial blood finds its way into the vein defect and a path of least resistance is established. A marked continuous thrill is felt and a corresponding continuous bruit is heard. The local venous system undergoes dilatation and varicosities may develop. The more proximal the fistula the greater is the likelihood of eventual high output cardiac failure.

Effects of injury

Blood loss

Rapid haemorrhage from a large vessel can result in exsanguination and death. In those who survive, the sequence of blood and fluid loss, depletion of circulation volume, hypotension and shock culminates in reduced tissue perfusion and anoxia. This situation will further endanger the organ or extremity to which blood flow has already been cut off by the vascular injury itself.

Coagulation defects

Haemorrhage, especially if torrential, results in loss of platelets and specific clotting factors, problems which can be compounded by massive transfusion of stored blood.

Renal failure

Prolonged hypotension following blood loss and either delayed or inadequate replacement and resuscitation may lead to renal failure. Crush injury or extensive ischaemia of limbs may cause acute tubular necrosis. External evidence of crush injury may be limited to signs of bruising or a fracture. Necrosis of muscle cells releases myoglobin and other breakdown products which block the renal tubules and cause acute tubular necrosis, particularly when renal blood flow is decreased.

A patient with the crush syndrome remains anxious for two or three days and then becomes drowsy, begins to vomit and complains of thirst, later becoming delirious as uraemia supervenes. He remains hypotensive and develops peripheral vasoconstriction and oliguria. Examination of blood will reveal a raised haematocrit, hyperkalaemia, raised urea and creatinine, while urine will contain albumin and dark casts. Anuria soon develops and prognosis is poor without renal dialysis.

Limb ischaemia

A period of ischaemia increases capillary permeability, interstitial pressure and venous pressure. Muscle fibres deprived of blood for more than four to eight hours become oedematous and, being confined within fascial compartments, are rendered more ischaemic. This swelling is aggravated by haematoma, vein injury or soft tissue trauma. Muscle fibres die after a maxium period of six to eight hours total occlusion and therefore speed of revascularization is essential. The oedema which follows restoration of flow raises intracompartmental pressure further, aggravating the ischaemia and even obliterating the main arteries.

Muscle contracture

Volkmann's ischaemic contracture occurs rarely after fractures. The classic example is seen in children who sustain fractures at the elbow, especially of the supracondylar type. Persistent arterial spasm or direct arterial injury may cause aseptic muscle necrosis of flexor muscles of the forearm which are replaced by fibrous tissue. A similar outcome may affect the calf muscles after superficial femoral or popliteal artery injury, whether closed or open.

Infection

Infection is a potential complication of penetrating trauma especially when contamination is at its greatest, i.e., resulting from high-velocity missiles and bombs. Failure to employ antibiotics, delayed and inadequate surgical toilet of the wound, delayed or defective vascular repair, the use of prosthetic grafts or premature wound closure will each contribute to this complication. Established infection may give rise to life-endangering secondary haemorrhage. Organisms cultured in these wounds cover a whole range of gram positive cocci and gram negative bacilli. In areas of muscle necrosis and where oedematous muscle is exposed following transcutaneous fasciotomy, *Pseudomonas aeruginosa* may be a tenacious pathogen.

Gas gangrene

Gas gangrene or clostridial myositis may complicate ischaemic injury, especially after inadequate exploration, limited debridement and wound toilet. Prevailing anaerobic conditions with reduced oxygen tension will allow spore regeneration. Tissues exhibit tense oedema and crepitus advancing rapidly upwards along muscle planes with brick-red discoloration of necrotic muscle. These developments are accompanied by toxaemia and cardiovascular collapse.

Amputation

Immediate. Extensive irreversible damage by the wounding agent will result in immediate amputation. In such cases delay may invite the very real dangers of infection, gas gangrene, secondary haemorrhage and renal failure which can be fatal.

Later. Late amputation may be the ultimate sequel to the following conditions: delayed arrival and exploration, ligation of vessels, inadequate repair, untimely fasciotomy and infection.

Air embolism

Air embolism may be associated with a vein laceration and carries special significance in cervical injuries. Discovery of such an injury, especially of the jugular vein, requires an expeditious head-down tilt of the table to decrease the risk of air embolism.

Chemical injury

Accidental intra-arterial injection of thiopentone into the arm may immediately produce severe burning pain, intense pallor and later give rise to skin discoloration, muscle contracture and gangrene.

The changes in pH of thiopentone on mixing with arterial blood results in the precipitation of solid crystals of thiopentone which block arterioles and capillaries. In addition, the drug provokes local release of large quantities of catecholamines with subsequent intense circulatory shutdown. However, intra-arterial thrombosis is the essential lesion which leads to tissue death.

VASCULAR INJURIES OF LIMBS

Early Management

Emergency treatment to be carried out would be:
1 *Control bleeding.* Firmly applied gauze pads and pressure bandages

are usually adequate to control external bleeding. If this method is ineffectual then a vascular clamp ought to be used in preference to a haemostat, which crushes the vessel wall and leads to needless further excision. Blind application of clamps in deep wounds may damage vessels or nerves.

2 *Restore loss.* Standard energetic resuscitative measures including oxygenation must be instituted. Hypotension, if prolonged, will compound the ischaemia of vascular injury. Blood, usually warmed and microfiltered, is transfused using O Rhesues negative in emergencies. Plasma substitutes and expanders are administered only in cases of shock. Resuscitation using matched whole blood is continued during operation.

3 *Medication.* Prophylactic tetanus toxoid and broad-spectrum antibiotics are indicated for cases of vascular trauma. If the patient is not hypotensive, narcotic analgesics are useful as they decrease vasospasm and serve as anaesthetic premedication.

4 *History.* Try to establish the tme of injury and therefore the interval before admission. What was the nature of the wounding agent? If a gun was used, was it of low or high muzzle velocity? What was the estimated amount of blood lost?

5 *Examination.* A brisk clinical examination should be done to locate external bleeding and to control it effectively. In a case of multiple injuries involving different disciplines, the appropriate surgical teams are notified immediately.

(a) *The wound.* Look at the affected limb and run through a check list, asking yourself the following questions. If bleeding is persistent, is it arterial, venous or mixed? If a haematoma is present, is it pulsatile or expanding? Is there a thrill or audible bruit indicating an acute arteriovenous fistula?

(b) *Distal flow.* Are pulses felt in vessels distal to the injury — the radial and ulnar in the upper limb and the posterior tibial, dorsalis pedis and peroneal in the lower limb? Remember that palpable pulse must not be construed as evidence of integrity of the proximal vessel. The detection of audible Doppler signals and the type of pulse waveform will assist in diagnosis. Note pallor, mottling, coolness, oedema and muscle tenderness. Tests employing capillary or venous filling are unreliable in arterial injury.

(c) *Spasm.* A diagnosis of spasm should not be made except at operation, if necessary excluding an intimal tear by performing an arteriotomy. This in particular applies to traction or stretch injury following blunt trauma; the absence of overt bleeding and the presence of apparently adequate collateral blood flow when pulses cannot be felt may lead to the erroneous inference that spasm is responsible.

(d) *Associated injury.* Is a neurological deficit present? Loss of sensation of glove or boot distribution may simply be due to ischaemia of motor nerves may cause muscle paralysis. Clinical evidence of associated bone and joint injury should be looked for. When fractures are associated with ischaemia, arterial injury and occlusion rather than spasm and external pressure may be responsible and should be given immediate consideration so as to avoid delays in instituting proper treatment.

Radiological investigations

Plain X-rays

In non-urgent cases, X-rays are taken to identify bony injury and to locate bullets or foreign bodies so that the correct incision can be made. Although plain films are of assistance in 'missile-tracking' they may have to be dispensed with, as delay in the radiology department, particularly in major vessel injury, can be dangerous and even fatal.

Angiography

Preoperative angiography must be selective. It may waste time in a clinically obvious injury, does not necessarily exclude venous injury, and is sometimes unreliable in revealing existing injury. However, each case must be judged on its own merits and rigid rules are not tenable. In certain circumstances, for instance when arterial injury is suspected despite the presence of palpable distal pulses, angiography will clarify the picture. When casualties arrive late or are transferred from other hospitals and have to be assessed afresh, then angiography can be of significant assistance if performed immediately. Biplanar angiography may expose an otherwise undetectable injury of the popliteal artery.

Operative management

Emergency amputation

When a limb is mutilated beyond repair, it is better to complete the amputation at a level of evident tissue viability. An attempt should be made to preserve as much healthy tissue as possible for delayed closure on which occasion the flaps can be tailored to create a satisfactory stump.

Incisions

In cases of lower limb injuries, both legs are prepared to enable removal of a donor vein from the uninjured limb. Classical longitudinal incisions are employed in the approach to vessels of upper and lower limbs. These incisions may have to be modified in cases of penetrating injury. In the case of popliteal vessels a gentle S-shaped posterior incision is preferred as it provides wider exposure distally. Adequate exposure and control of vessels above the site of injury is necessary, particularly when the common femoral artery is involved.

Exploration and preparation of vessels

The injured vessels are quickly exposed and controlled proximally and distally by vascular clamps, leaving 1–2 cm of vessel on either side of the injury which can then be trimmed back to a point where the whole vessel wall, including the intima is intact.

Exploration of vessels in each direction by means of Fogarty balloon catheters will often recover clot, especially when back bleeding is poor or absent. These catheters, properly and delicately used are invaluable; in inexperienced hands they can cause severe damage to otherwise normal vessels. Vigorous upward milking of the limb musculature distal to the injury will also express recent clot. Proximal and distal vessels are then perfused with heparinised saline (5000 units of heparin in 250 ml saline). In the absence of other injuries systemic heparinization is reliable.

Intraluminal shunting of vessels

In recent years, in order to restore arterial flow urgently and thereby reduce ischaemia time and arrest or minimize tissue damage, the author has used intraluminal shunts of the type employed in carotid artery surgery. These are introduced as soon as the vessel ends have been trimmed. As collateral flow is excellent following subclavian and axillary artery injury, shunting is really not required for these vessels.

In addition to revitalizing the distal limb, the use of such a shunt in a damaged adjacent vein should prevent serious oedema and a dangerous rise in intracompartmental pressure. In most instances fasciotomy was avoided without complication. In the presence of an associated fracture the shunt has the added advantage of allowing bony fixation to be accomplished effectively and without undue haste before commencing vascular repair. Donor vein grafts can be drawn over the shunt, which acts as a stent facilitating completion of most of the anastomotic suturing before it is removed.

In the event of admission of a patient who has sustained multiple injuries, limb-threatening vascular trauma can be left with such shunts *in situ*, thus buying time to enable life-endangering surgery to be completed first.

Wound care and debridement

Exploration of all penetrating wounds is recommended if disasters are to be avoided. It should be remembered in bullet wounds that missile velocity and the extent of tissue damage cannot be estimated reliably from the mere scrutiny of entrance and exit wounds. Skin around these wounds is excised sparingly. Devitalized muscle, recognized by its dark purplish colour and failure to bleed or contract, must be trimmed back to a point where it bleeds. The fascia should be incised liberally to allow free drainage thereby preventing intracompartmental compression. Free bony fragments, foreign bodies and other contaminants which may be deeply embedded are removed and the wound is copiously irrigated. Nerves in the vicinity of the vascular injury are carefully inspected; the degree of injury is noted and if significant marked with a silk suture for future reference.

Artery injury

The type of vascular repair indicated will depend on the injury. Vessels are trimmed with sharp arterial scissors. Fine, smooth, atraumatic polypropylene which is inert and possesses great tensile strength is the ideal suture material. A continuous everting suture is acceptable for large vessels but in those vessels less than 4 mm diameter, interrupted sutures are preferred to avoid constriction.

1 *Lateral suture.* A vessel laceration may permit lateral suture as long as, in doing so, the diameter of the lumen is not reduced and only after ascertaining the absence of intimal damage beyond the margins of the laceration. Lateral suture is rarely justified in arteries such as the

popliteal where the quality of repair is of critical importance.

2 *Patch angioplasty.* In order to preserve vessel calibre, angioplasty using a vein patch is preferable to lateral suture of a defect in the wall. This defect may be the direct consequence of injury or may follow trimming of a ragged laceration.

3 *Direct anastomosis.* Direct end-to-end repair is rarely feasible and is unjustified if the joint has to be flexed, however slightly, or if collateral channels have to be sacrificed to permit approximation. For these reasons, excision of a damaged vessel segment followed by vein grafting is preferred.

4 *Vein graft.*

(a) *Preparation of host artery.* The use of interposition vein grafts permits adequate excision of damaged wall; the dangers of breakdown bleeding and thrombosis which follow end-to-end anatomosis under tension are also avoided. The external appearances of an injured artery often belie the extent of internal damage. Beyond the obviously torn intima, the apparently undisturbed luminal surface may reveal microscopic evidence of endothelial loss, breaks in the elastic membrane, subintimal haemorrage and microthrombus formation. When in doubt the vessel should be opened and trimmed back ot a point where the intima is intact.

(b) *Donor vein.* The long saphenous vein of the opposite limb is the ideal souce for a vein graft. It is important to avoid using the ipsilateral vein because venous drainage to the whole leg may be compromised by the presence of concomitant deep vein injury. Donor vein is stored temporarily in Hank's solution or heparinized saline.

(c) *Type of vein graft.* The vein graft may be reversed and used as a simple interposition graft. Alternatively, it may be fashioned into a larger diameter graft by taking two segements of vein which are then opened longitudinally. These two panels are sewn together side by side to form a compound graft achieving a diameter comparable to that of the host vessel, thus ensuring laminar flow.

5 *Prosthetic graft.* The indiscriminate use of prosthetic grafts for missile-induced vascular trauma is ill-advised, except for arteries like the common femoral or larger. Such grafts are vulnerable to infection and secondary haemorrhage, as well as to the constant strain on anastomoses when they are placed at or near joints such as the knee.

6 *False aneurysm.* A false aneurysm must be removed. If saccular, it is excised at the neck and the defect closed by lateral suture or by patch angioplasty. If larger and fusiform, segmental excision and replacement with an interposed vein graft is better.

7 *Arteriovenous fistula.* The artery and vein are exposed, brought under control and the communication is divided. The openings in both artery and vein can be repaired successfully either by lateral suture or by insertion of a vein patch.

Cover

It is important to ensure adequate cover of vessels by adjacent tissues. If much tissue is lost then it is permissble to swing over unessential neighbouring muscles such as the sartorius and gracilis. Open wound drainage is preferable to vacuum suction drainage. The wound is covered with loose non-adherent absorbent dressings and left open for delayed primary suture or skin grafting 5–7 days later. Primary closure invites infection, the most alarming variety being gas gangrene. This latter dangerous complication may follow inadequate exploration and injudicious closure of wounds, especially those situated in the buttock, groin and upper thigh.

Vein injury

As with arterial injuries, ligation of injured veins should be avoided as far as possible. Every effort should be made to repair the common femoral and popliteal veins. A vein tolerates lateral suturing much better than an artery but loss of diameter must still be guarded against. Following vein injury at least one major channel of satisfactory calibre must be restored to avoid a rise in peripheral venous resistance and pressure. This can reduce arterial inflow and either promote thrombosis at the site of an arterial repair with consequent gangrene, or lead to chronic oedema with post-thrombotic changes.

In combined arterial and venous injury, preliminary vein repair allows arterial reconstruction to be carried out in a dry field, and free venous drainage prevents a serious rise in venous pressure once arterial flow is re-established. If intraluminal shunts are used in both artery and vein, the order of repair no longer becomes a subject for debate.

Fasciotomy

Why? The oedema which follows restoration of flow further raises intracompartmental pressure and the later the repair the more significant this factor becomes. Fasciotomy is therefore of paramount importance. A fasciotomy which is delayed and conservative inceases the chances of amputation, particularly after popliteal vessel injury.

When? This procedure is necessary if any one of the following is present: sustained hypotension, a period exceeding four hours between injury and revascularization, obvious muscle oedema noted at operation, concomitant artery and vein injury, significant bony injury, and finally, marked distal soft tissue trauma arising either from a closed crush injury or from an open high-velocity missile wound.

How? The classical percutaneous method of three compartment fasciotomy is employed as rule, the anterior compartment lying within rigid confines being the most vulnerable. Care is taken to avoid damage to the external peroneal and sural nerves. If obvious tension is still present then the skin and subcutaneous tissues must also be incised. It should be remembered that there is a fourth deep compartment and all four of these can be decompressed after first resecting the mid-third of the shaft of the fibula for access.

Associated fractures

1 *Treat fracture first.* If an artery is simply compressed or displaced by bone, flow is restored by bone reduction and fixation. When fractures accompany vascular injury, it is advisable to stabilize bone before attempting vascular repair for fear of disrupting a delicate reconstruction during manipulation. However, ischaemia time is critical and until recently the necessary fixation had to be accomplished expeditiously. However, in recent years, personal experience of the routine insertion of intraluminal shunts in both injured artery and vein has permitted unhurried bony stabilization prior to vascular repair.
2 *Type of bone fixation.* Internal fixation is acceptable for closed injuries. With contaminated wounds, external fixation is preferred. Skeletal traction may compromise an arterial repair, but external fixation

using a Hoffmann's or Belfast fixator, or other similar system, has been quite successful.

3 *Plaster casts.* Plaster cast techniques such as quadrilateral ischial-bearing long leg cast for femoral fractures and the patellar tendon-bearing short leg cast for tibial fractures have, in the past, enhanced early mobilization and discharge from hospital. These casts must not be used until the wound has been closed by suture or skin grafting and only after swelling has subsided. If they are employed soon after injury then they must be applied over a liberal layer of wool bandage and should be split or bivalved. The serious risk of occluding vascular repairs or restricting venous or lymphatic flow by tight circumferential dressings and splints must be kept in mind.

Joints

Joint damage is not uncommon in penetrating injuries caused by bullets. A haemarthrosis may occur and is usually associated with a degree of articular damage. Bullets and metal must be removed to prevent continuing injury or chemical synovitis.

Chemical injury

If thiopentone or diazepam is injected into an artery, such as the brachial, the following immediate steps may be helpful. Without removing the needle responsible, the following drugs are injected through it: 20,000 units of heparin (anticoagulant), 40–80 mg of papaverine (vasodilator) in 10–20 ml saline, procaine hydrochloride (vasodilator) 10–20 ml of 0.5 per cent solution, tolazolone (noradrenaline antagonist) 5 ml of 1 per cent solution. A single large dose of methylprednisolone may help to stablize the endothelium and enhance vasodilatation. Prostacyclin, a newly discovered vasodilator and inhibitor of platelet aggregation, may also be of value.

The operation is abandoned if possible and a brachial plexus or stellate ganglion block is performed to remove vasoconstrictor influence. If larger vessels are thrombosed, they must be quickly explored to remove clot, and the procedure repeated as needed. Heparin, tolazolone and perhaps dextran 40 should be administered by continuous infusion. Intravenous therapy may be discontinued and replaced by warfarin or dipryridamole and soluble acetylsalicylates until maximum recovery has occurred.

Postoperative management

Position and warming

To counteract the cooling of prolonged exposure during surgery and the vasoconstriction resulting from arrested flow, the careful supervised use of a heat cradle for a short time can be very helpful, at the same time taking the precaution to protect the legs with a blanket. A limb with arterial injury is left horizontal unless oedema is excessive or if vein injury is also present in which case some elevation is justified. The upper limbs can be elevated on pillows or by means of a sling while the lower limbs are easily elevated by raising the foot of the bed. A bed cage is placed over the legs and the feet and pulses must be available for regular inspection.

Adjunctive treatment

Anticoagulation with low dose heparin (5000 units six–eight hourly subcutaneously) and the administration of low molecular weight dextran to aid vascular patency are permissible but best avoided if there is risk of bleeding from other injuries. Dextran is contra-indicated when renal function is impaired.

Observations

Postoperative vigilance is essential in monitoring peripheral pulses and skin circulartion. In the absence of palpable pulses, signals from a Doppler flow detector will substantiate a clinical impression of adequate collateral blood supply.

Graft failure

If suspicions of failure are aroused, angiography must be undertaken immediately to demonstrate defective repair or graft closure. Oedema and dusky discoloration in the presence of distal arterial pulses may indicate venous thrombosis. Re-exploration for thrombotic occlusion, whether of artery or vein, must be undertaken without delay. These graft failures are often due to insufficient excision of damaged vessels, or deficiencies in technique. Initial operative treatment by experienced vascular surgeons will reduce the need for re-exploration.

Later care

During the following days, nerve function, both motor and sensory, should be checked and the power of individual muscle groups recorded. Wounds must be dressed daily or more frequently and wound swabs cultured. All vital signs including temperature and urinary output are monitored. If the crush syndrome is likely then renal function is carefully scrutinized.

Appropriate physiotherapy is essential during the recovery period both in hospital and later, on an outpatient basis, especially if the effects of nerve injury, e.g., a foot drop, have to be countered. Nerve conduction studies will establish a baseline, particularly when one is unsure whether muscle dysfunction has resulted from neurogenic or ischaemic injury. In cases of associated bony injury, orthopaedic and vascular surgeons should coordinate postoperative care.

Amputation

Amputation may become necessary if the patient arrives too late, if definitive vascular repair and fasciotomy are untimely or indequate, or if serious infection supervenes. The case histories of patients who require amputation illustrate the several pitfalls which confront the vascular surgeon.

ABDOMINAL VASCULAR INJURIES

Don't forget the thorax

The abdominal cavity extends from the level of the nipple line above to that of the gluteal crease below. Not surprisingly, about one quarter of penetrating abdominal wounds are accompanied by simultaneous involvement of the thoracic gravity. In diagnosis or management the abdominal cavity must not be considered in isolation. For example, failure to respond to vigorous fluid replacement prior to abdominal exploration or sudden deterioration in the absence of serious blood loss within the abdomen should signal the possibility of a missed cardio-pulmonary injury.

Assessment and initial care

The patient should be fully undressed to enable accurate examination and so that all penetrating wounds can be identified and the path of the wounding agent defined.

In closed injuries note the location of bruises and abrasions. Also look for the characteristic pattern bruising of seat belts, tyre marks or other objects which will point to crush injury of underlying organs. Pallor, a rising pulse rate and falling blood pressure may be signs of internal haemorrhage.

The patient's blood is typed and at least 10–12 units of whole blood crossmatched. Samples are taken for haematocrit, urea and electrolyte and Astrup estimations. Large venous access lines are inserted into uninjured veins fluid infusions and blood replacement. An airway is introduced if necessary and a nasogastric tube is passed. If time permits, X-rays of the chest and abdomen are taken to provide essential pointers to determine correct operative access.

Closed injuries

It is worthwhile emphasising in closed injuries that the presence of intra-peritoneal blood or urine may not abolish bowel sounds even when a hollow viscus has been perforated. Note abdominal girth and watch for increasing distension, particularly if the patient is unconscious and cannot complain of pain. Repeat examination of the abdomen related to frequent observation of vital signs is of inestimable value.

Penetrating injuries

In penetrating abdominal injuries exploration is mandatory irrespective of clinical findings. Abdominal distension and rapid deterioration alert one to the probability of injury to major vessel trunks. In these circumstances, X-rays and peritoneal lavage are futile investigations. There must be no delay in operating on these individuals as the situation becomes irretrievable very quickly.

Resuscitation

In some cases, the MAST (Military Anti Shock Trousers) or G-suit has been used successfully to control bleeding and to raise pressure while definitive surgery is begun.

In acute hypovolaemic shock, Ringer's lactate can be used in an emergency to replace almost half the blood volume. This brings the haematocrit to approximately 20 per cent which will temporarily provide acceptable oxygen transport. The patient remains hypotensive or, at best, shows only a transient response to intravenous infusions. In major trunk vessel injuries, therefore, operative control constitutes the one and only effective resuscitative procedure.

Emergency thoracotomy

It has been advocated that when a patient presents with a tense haemo-peritoneum and persistent hypotension, an urgent preliminary left thoracotomy and temporary clamping of the descending thoracic aorta prior to laparotomy will control haemorrhage, ensure continued perfusion of heart and brain and at laparotomy allow thorough examination of the upper abdomen.

Preoperative routine

The neck, chest, abdomen and thighs are prepared if time is available. An intact abdominal wall provides temporary tamponade which helps to limit continuing losses. This protection is eliminated first by deep anaesthesia and muscle relaxation and then by laparotomy. Light anaesthesia is advisable initially, and muscle relaxants are withheld until one is ready to enter the abdomen. This approach will prevent a perilous final drop on blood pressure.

Laparotomy

Unless the assumed path of the bullet dictates otherwise, a long mid-line incision gives access and good exposure in seriously ill patients. It allows thorough inspection and evaluation of the entire abdominal cavity and can be easily extended into the chest either by splitting the sternum or by anterolateral thoracotomy, depending on the organs one has to expose to best advantage.

Control of bleeding

The first priority must be the control of major bleeding, commonest cause of death in penetrating abdominal wounds. Torrential haemorrhage may follow laparotomy, hence large amounts of blood must be available in the operating theatre. The rapid evacuation of clots and delivery of bowel outside the abdominal cavity permits freer access for definition of injury both by sight and palpation. Blind application of forceps or vascular clamps may be dangerous and will cause further damage. Large packs are inserted firmly and then removed singly, dealing with each bleeding vessel in turn. Compression of the subdiaphragmatic aorta against the vertebral bodies by the heel of the hand or an aortic compressor can impede flow significantly until a clamp is applied.

Retroperitoneal haematoma

A retroperitoneal haematoma, especially if large and expanding, may conceal major vessel injury and must be carefully explored after proximal and distal control. Retroperitoneal injuries are particularly treacherous because damage to aorta and cava may coexist with serious injury to pancreas, duodenum, colon and urinary tract which may be missed until it is too late.

Repair of the aorta

Separate cross-clamps above and below an aortic laceration may not be as effective as large side-biting partial occlusion clamps. In the absence of bowel contamination classical methods of repair by means of lateral suture, patch grafting or interposition of a tube prosthesis are employed. Primary repair especially with a prosthesis may be compromised by coincidental bowel injury and faecal contamination. If aortic damage is extensive in such a case then the aorta may be oversewn and a temporary extra-anatomic bypass, namely, an axillo-bifemoral bypass, may have to be constructed.

The aorta being large will tolerate lateral suture. An anterior defect may be extended longitudinally to permit lateral suture of a posterior laceration from within. If the defect is too large, continuity is retained and a wide dacron patch graft is inserted. Alternatively, a short dacron tube graft is interposed. Access to suprarenal aortic injuries is more difficult and management is further complicated by renal, coeliac and superior mesenteric vessel injury as well as by damage to the duodenum and pancreas. If necessary, combined partial pancreatectomy and splenectomy is permissible to enable reconstruction of the aorta. Reimplantation or repair of the renal arteries and the main visceral trunks is imperative if ischaemic infarction of the organs concerned is to be averted.

Repair of the vena cava

Every effort must be made to restore major venous channels. The cava can be controlled by a partial occlusion clamp to repair a laceration by lateral suture or vein patch. The infrarenal cava is exposed directly, after reflecting the small bowel mesentery to the right. When the infrarenal vena cava is badly torn by a high-velocity bullet, ligation is preferable to attempted repair in the midst of exsanguinating haemorrhage.

The suprarenal cava is exposed by Kocher's manoeuvre and reflection of the duodenum and head of pancreas to the right. This portion of the cava must be reconstituted, if necessary by means of a free graft from the infrarenal cava.

When the retrohepatic cava or hepatic veins are injured the right chest is opened, a pericardiotomy performed and a large calibre chest tube is inserted through a purse-string in the right atrium and guided down into the inferior vena cava. This tube is 'snugged' at the intrathoracic and suprarenal parts of the inferior vena cava thereby controlling haemorrhage but enabling adequate venous return to the heart.

Formal repair of the cava and hepatic veins behind the liver will usually necessitate a transhepatic approach.

Pelvic vessels

Bleeding from large pelvic vessels, especially veins, may be particularly troublesome to control. A common or external iliac artery injury should be reconstructed but the internal iliac artery can be safely ligated if haemorrhage is uncontrollable. Severe iliac vein damage is best dealt with by ligation.

Superior mesenteric and portal veins

After digital control by Pringle's method, i.e., by compressing the free border of the lesser omentum, the portal vein is exposed by Kocher's manoeuvre and repaired. The superior mesenteric vein is more easily exposed and reconstructed.

VASCULAR INJURIES IN THE NECK

The next contains a number of vital anatomical structures placed closely together and the management of injuries in this region is always a serious undertaking requiring considerable experience.

Cuffed endotracheal tube

In penetrating injuries the importance of immediate endotracheal intubation with a cuffed tube must be emphasised. This action will prevent extravasated blood from entering the lungs and also secure an airway in the presence of an expanding neck haematoma or tracheal injury. An assured airway will minimise anoxia–induced cerebral oedema. Athough bleeding from carotid and vertebral arteries and jugular vein can be massive, the control of haemorrhage is comparatively less important in these circumstances. The presence of an anaesthetist is desirable. If blood has entered the lungs, rapid suction of the bronchi is essential. Blunt injury or severe contusion by crushing or strangulaton may result in tense haematomas and vessel damage, dangerously threatening the airway. The passage of a nasogastric tube in th emergency room should be avoided because coughing and gagging may promote further haemorrhage.

Angiography

Should a patient arrive with developing neruological signs angiography becomes a luxury one cannot afford. Delayed restoration of flow may cause haemorrhagic infarction of the brain. If there is time and certainly if the injury is located at the root of the neck or base of skull, angiography will be of help in defining the type and extent of injury or in demonstrating, for example, if a carotico–jugular fistula is present.

Exploration

These wounds must be explored even though the patient is stable and the wound looks innocuous and shows no sign of bleeding. The morbidity of negative exploration is minimal but deadly complications may follow a conservative approach. Unexplored wounds have presented later with the serious complication of carotico–jugular fistula. In such cases the patient usually complains of a continuous loud noise in his ear.

Carotid arteries

Penetrating injury will result in severe external and internal bleeding while blunt injury or traction injury may cause an intimal tear with dissection, thrombotic occlusion and stroke. With early admission there is no reason why reconstruction of the common and internal carotid arteries should not be performed using an intraluminal shunt if necessary. While end-to-end repair of the common carotid is often possible, vein graft interposition would be indicated in most instances of internal carotid injury.

Vertebral arteries

These may bleed massively and are a potential source of cerebral ischaemia. Exposure and repair through the neck is difficult but can be facilitated by removing the medial half of the clavicle.

Jugular vein

The internal jugular vein ought to be repaired rather than ligated. When a torn jugular vein is noted and especially if it is empty, a head-down tilt of the table below the level if the heart must be quickly carried out to decrease the risk of air embolism. Simultaneously the open vessel is covered firmly and then controlled in preparation for repair.

Subclavian vessels

1 *Clinical presentation.* In injuries at the root of the neck the subclavian vessels are likely to be involved producing massive haemorrhage internally into the neck and chest, often also damaging elements of the brachial plexus. Occasionally the apex of the lung may be damaged giving rise to severe surgical emphysema.

2 *First part.* The first part of the right subclavian artery is best approached through a median sternotomy which also allows control of all the great vessels. This incision can be extended into the neck if necessary. The first part of the left subclavian artery is best exposed by adding a high anterior thoracotomy at the third or fourth rib with division of the clavicle so as to provide a 'trap-door' approach.

3 *Second part.* Access to the second part of the subclavian vessels, especially on the right side, may be gained by a supraclavicular incision extended to permit removal of the medical half of the clavicle.

4 *Third part.* In addition to external causes of injury, the part of the subclavian artery may be damaged by a fractured clavicle. The mid–third of the clavicle is removed to provide exposure.

5 *Ligation.* The rich collateral circulation around the subclavian causes profuse bleeding regardless of proximal control. This very collateral, however, will permit safe ligation of the second and third parts of the subclavian if primary repair is not feasible.

6 *Secondary haemorrhage.* Death may occur later from sudden torrential haemorrhage externally or into the pleural cavity, particularly with high-velocity bullet damage and infection. The likelihood of breakdown is enhanced by the absence of adequate soft tissue cover for these rather delicate vessels.

THE FUTURE

Future progress in this fairly damanding surgical discipline will rely heavily on a critical review of one's experience. Review and especially the long-term follow-up of patients, the assessment of graft patency and surgical complications, as well as research aimed at overcoming existing difficulties, together represent a continuing learning process. To achieve this goal it is important to keep an accurate record of the history of a vascular injury and the clinical findings noted, and meticulous documentation of the details of surgical treatment is essential. These notes will provide an invaluable source of data for someone analysing and reporting results.

Advances in the treatment of vascular injuries in Northern Ireland have been in part a product of local experience but in larger measure based on a foundation of lessons learned through decades of international military and civilian experience of vascular trauma.

19 Fractures in children

Children's bones are not as brittle as adults. Greenstick fractures occur when one cortex breaks and the other buckles. Minor fractures may only show as a slight bulge on the X-ray. The periosteum is relatively thicker — this restricts displacement in some long-bone fractures. Healing is more rapid and non-union is rare.

Diagnostic difficulty in interpreting X-rays is a hazard for the inexperienced. Epiphyseal plates may look like fractures, and comparison views of the uninjured side may be very helpful.

Ligaments are often stronger than epiphyseal plates, so dislocations are uncommon. With growth, remodelling can correct a malunion. The capacity to remodel decreases with advancing maturity and with distance of fracture from growing epiphysis. Remodelling occurs only in the line of the primary action of the adjacent joint.

When overgrowth occurs from hyperaemia of the limb stimulating epiphyseal activity, such overgrowth is permanent.

Specific injuries

Clavicular fractures

These are very common in children and initially no specific treatment other than wearing a sling for a few days is required if the joints at either end are not involved.

Epiphyseal separation of proximal humerus

Closed reduction is required only for severe displacements but remodelling is excellent and less severe injuries are treated in a sling or stockingette velpeua bandage. Open reduction is not justified, even with a poor reduction.

Supracondylar fracture of the humerus

This is a common injury in children under the age of eight years. It can be serious and must be thoroughly understood. By definition it occurs above the condyles and hence should not have damaged the growth plates. Almost all are displaced posteriorly and are, therefore, treated in flexion.

The neurological and vascular status of the limb must be examined at the earliest opportunity. Recording the radial pulse and capillary return under the nails is not adequate examination of the circulation. The fingers and wrist of the conscious child must be gently extended and this should not cause further pain unless the circulation to the forearm muscles is compromised. Volkmann's ischaemic contracture is the name of the disabling stiff claw-like hand which results from necrosis and subsequent fibrosis of muscles. It is preventable. A useful mnemonic is the well know six P's: Pain, Pallor, Paralysis, Pulselessness, Paraethesia, Persisting Cold.

Any combination of the three main nerves around the elbow may be damaged — often neuropraxia only, but sometimes axonotemesis. The prognosis is good and, therefore, early exploration of the nerves is not usually indicated. The median nerve is most often damaged. The most sensitive test of its function is to examine flexion of the distal interphalangeal joint of the index finger and sensation over the pulp.

Treatment

Reduction under general anaesthetic may be required. Gross swelling may occur rapidly and make reduction difficult. If unsuccessful and particulary if there is concern for the circulation or sensation, modified Dunlop traction, i.e. straight arm traction, is a satisfactory, safe method of treatment. This allows daily examination of the carrying angle and avoidance of the late complication of cubitus varus. Rotatory, varus or valgus deformities cannot be expected to remodel. For late cubitus varus a supracondylar osteotomy may be required.

Fracture of the lateral condyle

This is common in small children. It can be very difficult to diagnose. Local tenderness and bruising are helpful signs. Radiographs of the other elbow may be useful. It is an injury involving the epiphyseal plate and, if displaced, requires open reduction and internal fixation.

Fracture of the medial epicondyle of the humerus

This fracture with displacement within the elbow joint may require open reduction. It can occur with dislocation of the elbow.

Fracture of the neck of the radius

This causes tilting of the head. Closed or open reduction may be necessary but the radial head must never be excised. Radiographs of the elbow sometimes fails to show any fracture. Pain and restriction of movement are probably caused by a haemoarthrosis but the joint must be rested until all irritability has subsided.

Fracture of the base of proximal phalanx of a finger

Problems can arise if it is not reduced. Malunion can lead to rotatory deformity. The digit should, therefore, be immobilised in flexion and pointing towards the insertion of flexor carpi radialis. Mobilisation of the finger should be started in about ten days.

Fractures of the femoral neck

These are very rare in children but have the same nasty complications as in adults. Internal fixation using smooth Newman's pins is often supplemented by a period in traction or plaster of Paris Hip Spica. Parents should be warned of the possible complications including avascular necrosis and growth arrrest.

Fractures of the shaft of the femur

These need accurate reduction if the child is over eleven years old. If under this age a slight overlap is acceptable because of the risk of overgrowth in younger children. Small children can be managed in Gallows (Bryant's) traction. Over the age of three, if they are unconscious or incontinent due to spinal injury or myelomeningocoele, they should be treated in balanced Hamilton Russell traction. Other children can be managed in a Thomas' splint using fixed traction and careful daily checks on leg length for the first two weeks.

Dislocations

In children the epiphyseal plate is often weaker than the ligaments and capsules around the joint, so dislocations are uncommon. However, they can occur at the hip, elbow or fingers. They should be reduced as soon as possible by closed means.

Epiphyseal injuries

Growth plates distinguish a child from an adult and an injury to a growing area may cause interference with growth. It is important that these injuries be assessed thoroughly, not only for correct treatment, but also so that the prognosis can be anticipated and parents advised accordingly. The Salter-Harris classification is recommended:

Type 1. Shearing of the epiphysis and its growth plate from the metaphysis. This injury commonly occurs by an inversion force to the ankle causing separation of the distal fibular epiphysis. It is frequently misdiagnosed as a sprain of the lateral ligament.

Type 2. In addition to Type 1, a triangular fragment is separated from the metaphysis. The distal radius is frequently damaged in falls on the outstretched hand and, in children, displacement of the epiphysis and growth plate is often accompanied by a metaphyseal fracture.
Types 1 and 2 have a good prognosis.

Type 3. The fracture line passes through the epiphysis into the joint and not through the metaphysis. This less common injury is sometimes seen at the ankle, involving the distal tibial epiphysis.

Type 4. The fracture line crosses through the epiphysis and the metaphysis. Lateral condylar fractures of the humerus are often obliquely across both metaphysis and epiphysis.
In types 3 and 4 accurate reduction is essential and this often requires open reduction and internal fixation. Growth arrest and deformity may occur.

Type 5. Compression injury to the epiphyseal plate which may be difficult to diagnose initially. Reversal of damage may be impossible. If a bony bridge occurs across the epiphyseal plate it may be possible to excise it if it is not too large. This uncommon injury is usually seen in the leg when the child falls from a height.
The prognosis should be guarded in Types 3, 4 and 5.

20 Open fractures

These are frequently referred to as compound fractures. A wound is present which communicates with the fracture. This may have been caused by the broken end of the bone piercing the skin from within or by pentration by an object from without. Greater violence has usually been involved. Open fractures are more serious because of the risk of infection. It is important to appreciate that any wound is at least contaminated by bacteria and possibly by other foreign material such as clothing or soil. Always check for neurovascular deficit as the wound may involve other soft tissues. Degloving, crush injury or tissue loss make the injury potentially more serious. In gunshot wounds establish whether the injury has been caused by high- or low-velocity missiles.

Treatment

The wound should be inspected briefly to ascertain the site and extent of the wound and whether bone is visible or not. After inspection a sterile dressing should be applied. Gross deformity is gently corrected and temporary splintage is applied. X-rays are taken and tetanus prophylaxis must be ensured. Prophylactic antibiotics are controversial but if they are to be given they should be given immediately. Much more important than prophylactic antibiotics is early radical debridement of the wound leaving only healthy bleeding tissue. Ideally this should be carried out within six hours of injury if possible. The original wound may have to be extended and enlarged to allow for adequate debridement. If there is any doubt the wounds should be left open. Delayed primary suture can be carried out five–six days later. Skin grafting may be necessary. If the fracture can be reduced and is stable a well padded plaster can be applied. This should be split to allow for postoperative swelling. External fixation devices are being used more and more to maintain reduction in these fractures. This also allows for wound inspection, secondary suture and skin grafting.

All gunshot wounds must be left open initially. Soft tissue damage is much greater in high- than in low-velocity injuries, consequently a more radical debridement is generally necessary. As there is often gross comminution of the bone an external fixation device is often very helpful in order to stabilize the fracture.

Postoperatively the limb is elevated. The patient's general condition and the condition of the limb should be observed frequently. Excessive pain should be investigated as it may mean that there is some degree of ischaemia or infection present. Once the soft tissue parts are healed, the external fixation device, if it has been applied, can be removed, usually after four–five weeks, and a well fitting plaster cast applied. Bony union of the fracture is often slower in open than in closed fractures.

21 Burns

Definition

A burn injury is caused by the release of energy into the tissues and may be due to heat, chemicals, electricity, radiation or friction singly or in combination. Individuals particularly at risk are the very young and the very old, people suffering from periods of unconsciousness and those working in hazardous occupations.

Assessment of injury

This involves the estimation of the depth and area of the burn. In relevant circumstances the possibility of a smoke inhalation injury should be considered.

Depth of burn

This is a consequence of the temperature of the burning agent and the duration of exposure to heat. Partial thickness burns are typically pink in colour and moist with some blistering. Pain sensitivity is preserved. Full thickness burns are typically dry and avascular in appearance and are insensitive to pinprick testing. Many of the deeper partial thickness burns may be difficult to classify but those which are initially unresponsive to pinprick testing should be grouped with full thickness injuries for the purpose of clinical management, as skin grafting is usually indicated to achieve rapid healing and minimal scarring. Many patients will, of course, have mixed areas of partial and full thickness injury.

The surface area of the burn

This is a major determining factor in the prognosis for survival, the others being the age of the patient, the presence of a lung injury and the pre-burn state of health. All areas of full and partial thickness burn are included but not areas of erythema. The rule of nines is applied where the head and neck and each of the upper limbs is nine per cent of total surface area and each surface of the trunk and each lower limb represent 18 per cent of total surface area. Adjustments are made for children, where the head is relatively larger and the lower limbs are relatively smaller.

Treatment of the burned skin

Small localised burns

Where these are partial thickness, outpatient treatment is often appropriate. The area should be covered by an occlusive dressing, sufficient in bulk to absorb the exudate and including an antibacterial cream. The dressing is changed about every three days, or sooner if the exudate has soaked through. Partial thickness burns of the hands are treated efficiently in polythene gloves, allowing independence and mobility of the hands during the healing period. If healing is not almost complete at twelve–fourteen days, consideration should be given to excision of the wound and skin graft cover. Small full thickness and deep dermal burns should be treated surgically at an early stage.

Larger burns

Inpatient treatment is usually more appropriate. The size of burn requiring admission will be influenced by the site of the injury and the patient's home conditions. Partial thickness burns may be treated by the exposure method when they involve only one body surface. Other partial thickness burns and all full thickness burns are better treated with occlusive dressings incorporating an antibacterial cream to reduce the risk of infection. Full thickness and deep partial thickness burns should be treated by wound excision and grafting commencing a few days after injury or when the patient is judged fit. In large burns the excision may need to be staged.

General management of the patient

Fluid resuscitation

A burn injury results in leakage of protein-rich fluid from the capillaries into the tissues, thus depleting the circulation. Oral fluid replacement is usually adequate for burns under 10 per cent in children and 15 per cent in adults. In more severe injuries intravenous resuscitation is appropriate. This aim is to anticipate the fluid loss and maintain a good circulating blood volume. The likely fluid requirements are estimated for periods ending four, eight, twelve, eighteen, twenty-four and thirty-six hours following injury. The estimated volume of fluid for each of these periods is given in ml. by the weight of the patient in kilogrammes multiplied by the percentage area burned over two. This fluid should be isotonic for salt and at least half given as plasma protein or substitute. The actual volume prescribed should be adjusted frequently to maintain a good hourly urinary output and a packed cell volume close to the normal range. A bladder catheter should be passed in patients with larger burns for accurate measurement of urine output.

Lung injury

This should be suspected in any patient burned in a fire in an enclosed space. It is due to chemical irritation. Blood gases should be measured. Treatment is with oxygen-enriched and humidified air and frequent physiotherapy (in more severe cases assisted ventilation will be required).

Pain relief

Strong analgesics must always be given intravenously during the resuscitation period.

Prevention of infection

Initial cultures are taken from the wounds and also the nose, throat and urine. Prophylactic antibiotics are not given except in cases of inhalation injury. Infection is prevented by good aseptic technique, effective anti-bacterial creams, and rapid closure of wounds with skin grafts.

Nutrition

The metabolic rate is very high. The patient's need for protein and energy must be met. In larger burns this usually means continuous feeding through a fine-bore nasogastric tube. It should be noted that patients with large injuries often have paralytic ileus in the initial stage of management.

Blood replacement

Blood transfusions should not be given during the resuscitation period but thereafter are necessary to maintain haemoglobin levels close to normal.

Fluid and electrolyte balance

Following resuscitation the patient may be quite oedematous. A liberal intake of salt-free fluids is required to allow excretion of the salt in the urine.

Physiotherapy

Bad position of joints must be avoided, if necessary making use of splints. As healing is achieved, joint movements are encouraged. Following healing of the burn there may be a long period of rehabilitation associated with maturation of the scars. Later surgery may be required for relief of joint contractures and other deformities.

22 Amputations and orthotics

Traumatic amputations

The level at which definitive amputation is performed has a life-long effect on the activity of the amputee. From below-knee to through-knee, and from below-elbow to through-elbow, is only a matter of inches, yet the difference in useful function is considerable. In traumatic amputations the circumstances for a thoughtful and careful elective procedure are rarely present. In these circumstances it is quite permissable to try and retain as much limb length as possible in the first place, and carry out the definitive amputation when the circumstances are better.

Immediate amputation

The normal surgical principles of surgical care apply. It may be that there is already a traumatic amputation with more proximal damage, or there may be a grossly damaged and non-viable limb. The normal debridement procedures are carried out with vigorous cleansing and excision of non-viable muscle, bone and other tissues. The danger of infection also dictates the need to leave the wound open initially, and secondary suture carried out a few days later. Whilst the question of definitive skin flaps is important, at the initial operation there should be every attempt to retain viable skin, for unconventional flaps may be needed when definitive amputation is carried out. There is also a tendency for skin flaps to retract, thus a few loose holding sutures are useful, especially to hold skin over exposed bone. In the heat of the moment, the surgeon should remember that the aim is to provide a 'useful' stump, as opposed to a surgically cosmetic stump.

At delayed primary suture, after a few days, there is an opportunity to tidy up the stump and apply skin grafts to bare areas. At this stage advice from a surgeon experienced in amputation surgery, or a doctor experienced in limb fitting could be of help.

Delayed definitive amputation

In order to retain length and produce a useful stump, procedures such as rotation flaps or further grafting may be necessary, with due account taken of areas that bear weight. The bone and muscle may have to be trimmed.

Amputation levels

There are optimal amputation levels, arrived at by a combination of factors, including stump viability and limb design.

Partial foot amputations. Many are described, but few are satisfactory, and most result in a painful equinus foot due to imbalance caused by the powerful Tendo Achilles. Toe amputations are reasonably successful, but Chopart's and Lisfranc's amputations would not be so popular were the surgeon able to follow them up.

Symes amputation. Provides a useful end-bearing stump, for which a good artificial limb can be provided.

Below-knee amputation. The retention of the knee joint and a variety of good prostheses give good functional results.

Through-knee amputation. The provision of a 'long lever' and some end-bearing, plus a new breed of prosthetic knee joints make this a reasonable amputation level, especially in the elderly.

Above-knee amputation. Usually a 'last resort' level, which should be avoided if a lower level can be achieved.

Arm Amputations. The lowest level possible is usually indicated.

Post-operative care

There is little point in producing an adequate amputation stump if the proximal joint is stiff or contracted. The staff should avoid propping up stumps with pillows and allowing long periods of joint flexion when sitting. The physiotherapist should also prevent contractures and build up wasted muscles. Oedema may be controlled by stump bandaging, and the stump shaped, and the patient taught how to carry out the procedure. Plans should also be made for the patient's return home with attention to social and vocational rehabilitation.

Orthotics

Immediate splintage

Plaster of Paris has the advantage of familiarity and cheapness, and is the traditional material to use to immobilise fractures. However, disadvantages include its weight, breakage if it becomes wet, and slowness in setting. To answer these disadvantages, several new materials have come on the market, and these include:

Baycast. A polyurethane resin with a muddy brown colour. It is very light and strong, is cured in five minutes, and the patient can bear weight in 30 minutes. Ideal for elderly patients, but is slightly inflammable, and is twice the cost of plaster of Paris.

Crystona. A mixture of acrylic polymer and aluminosilicate powder. Similar to plaster of Paris, but is sticky, and gloves or barrier cream should be used. It is slow to cure, but is strong and porous and is excellent as a waterproof layer over conventional plaster.

Hexalite. A wide meshed thermoplastic which softens in water at 70°C. Very useful for temporary pylons and splints, but considerably more expensive than Plaster of Paris.

Neofract. This is a type of polyurethane foam, produced by mixing two liquids. This mixture is spread between two layers of a cotton stocking, which is wrapped around the appropriate part. The cotton layer may have zip-fasteners attached, which allows the cast to be conveniently taken off. It is strong, light and water resistant, but its preparation is cumbersome, and it is costly.

Fracture bracing

Advances in orthotics, with the availability of new plastics, and strong lightweight joints, have produced a resurgence of interest in fracture bracing. Fracture bracing avoids the possible complications of operative fixation, and in femoral fractures reduces inpatient time from an average of fifteen weeks to an average of seven weeks. There are advantages also in early joint mobilisation. Time of union is similar in both fracture bracing and continuous traction and the incidence of non-union is similar.

Success in femoral fractures depends on adequate lateral pressure on the thigh cuff, to counteract displacement at the fracture site. It is also essential to maintain firm contact, and the plastic thigh cuff allows adjustment as the swelling diminishes.

Index

Abdominal injuries 26–31
  closed 26–31
    different types 26
    visceral damage 26–7
  penetrating 31
  vascular injuries 123–8
    aorta repair 126–7
    assessment and initial care 124
    bleeding control 126
    closed injuries 124
    pelvic vessels 127
    penetrating injuries 125
    vein repairs 127–8
Accident, main immediate tasks 3
Achilles tendon, rupture 95
Acromio-clavicular joint, dislocation 73
Adrenaline injection 51
Air embolism 113
Airway clearance 8–9
  in facial injuries 10
Amputations
  delayed definitive 142–3
  immediate 142
  levels 143–4
  post-operative care 143
  traumatic 142
  and vascular injury 113, 115–19, 123
    artery injury 117–19
    cover by tissues 119
    emergency 115–16
    intraluminal shunts 116–17
    vein injury 119
    wound care 117
Analgesia 47–9, 52
  inhalation 47–8
  parenteral 48–9
Anaphylactic shock 51
Aneurysm, false 110, 118
Angiography
  in head injury 10
  in neck injuries 128–9
  in vascular injury 115
Angioplasty, patch 118
Ankle fractures 95–6
Antibiotics 49–50, 52
  in fractures in children 20
  as prophylaxis 49–50
  in vascular injuries 112, 114
Anti-epileptics 51, 52
Anti-tetanus prophylaxis 48–9, 51
Anxiolytics 51, 52
Aorta, repair 126–7

Arm injuries 44–6
  see also Hand injuries; Limb injuries;
    Wrist
Arteriovenous fistula 110, 119
Artery injury, management 117–19
  see also Vascular injuries and specific
    names
Axonotemesis 46, 133

Barotrauma 70
Baycast 144
Biceps, long head, rupture 75
Bladder
  care in neurological injury 18–19
  rupture 39
    extraperitoneal 40–1
    intraperitoneal 39–40
Bleeding 278
  control 113–14
    in abdominal injuries 126
  drowning, and suffocation in chest
    injuries 21
  see also Haemorrhage
Blood
  loss 111
  pressure, monitoring 57
  transfusions 31
    in burns 141
  vessels, abdominal 30–1
Blow-out fractures, orbit 67–8
Blunt injury to vessels 108
Bowel rupture 29–30
Bronchus, ruptured 23
Burns
  conjunctiva 63–4
    chemical 63–4
  eyelid 62
  management 138–41
    assessment 138–9
    fluid resuscitation 139–40, 141
    infection 140
    lung injury 140
    nutrition 140–1
    physiotherapy 141
    treatment 139

Cardiac output, monitoring 58
Cardiovascular haemodynamics 56–8
Carotid arteries, injuries 129
Carpal bone dislocation 81
Catheters causing injuries to vessels 108
Central nervous system, monitoring 58

Index

Central venous pressure, monitoring 57
Cerebrospinal fluid leakage, ear 70
Cervical spine injuries 17-19
Chemical injuries to vessels 109, 113
Chest injuries 20-25
  closed 20-24
    bleeding, drowning and suffocation 21
    first aid management 21-2
    initial hospital management 22-3
    intrathoracic haemorrhage 23
    loss of lung function 20
    ruptured diaphragm 24
    ruptured trachea and bronchus 23
    treatment 20
  penetrating 25
Clavicle, fractures 73, 132
Coagulation defects 111
Collar bone fractures 73
Colles' fracture 80, 81
Compound fractures, treatment 136-7
Computerised tomography in head injury 10
Conjunctiva, injuries 63-4
Consciousness level, deterioration, in head injuries 9-10
Cornea
  abrasions 65
  lacerations 64
Corneo-scleral lacerations 65
Crush injuries to vessels 109
Crystona 144
Cyclimorph 49
Cyclizine 49

Dextran 122
Diaphragm, ruptured 24
Diazepam 51
  intra-arterial injection 109
  management 120-1
Dislocations 45, 76, 134
Drugs
  intra-arterial injection 109, 113, 120-1
  treatment 47-51

Ear, injuries 69-70
  cauliflower, preventing 69
  foreign bodies 72
  inner 70
  outer 69
Elbow, injuries to and around 76-8

Elbow, injuries to and around — *cont.*
  dislocation 76
  fractures 76-8
Electrocardiography 57
Endotracheal tube, cuffed, in neck injuries 128
Entonox 47-8, 52
Epicondylitis 78
Epilepsy control 51, 52
Epiphyseal injuries 78
  femoral 90-2
    fractures, in children 135-6
    slipped under 90
Epistaxis 71
Erb's palsy 73
Eye injuries 64-6
  contusions 66
  foreign bodies 66
  perforating 65-6
Eyelid injuries 61-2
  avulsion 62
  burns 62
  lacerations 61-2

Facial injuries 10-16
  mandible 12
  middle third 11-12
    fractures 12-13
  nerve 70
  position of patient 10
  resuscitation 5
  soft tissue injuries 16
  surgical anatomy 11
  zygoma fractures 14, 16
Fasciotomy 120
Fat embolism 58
Femur, fractures 85-7
  bracing 144-5
  in children 134-5
  shafts 102-3
Fibula and tibia, fractures 103
First aid in chest injuries 21-2
Foot, injuries 97-100
  fractures 97-100
Foreign bodies
  conjunctival 63
  corneal 64-5
  ear, nose and throat 72
  intra-ocular 66
Fractures 45
  associated with vessel injury 120-1
  bracing 144-5

Index

Fractures — *cont.*
  in children 132–5
  open, treatment 136–7
  see also specific bones

G-suit 125
Gas gangrene 112–13
Grafts, vein 118–19
  failure 122–3
Gunshot wounds, management 136–7

Haemaccel 5
Haematoma
  ear 69
  following injury 109
  nose 70
  retroperitoneal 126
Haemodynamics, cardiovascular 56–8
Haemorrhage
  control 5, 113–14
    in abdominal injuries 27–8, 126
    intrathoracic, and chest injuries 23
    rapid 111
    secondary 130
    subjunctival 63
Hand injuries 83–4
  bone and joint 84
  fractures 84
  nerves 83
  rehabilitation 84
  skin 83
  tendons 83
Hartmann's solution 5
Head injuries 8–16
  airway clearance 8–9
  deterioration of consciousness 9
  priorities 8–9
  recovery factor 8
  skull, investigations 9
  see also Facial injuries; Neck injuries
Heparin, low-dose 122
Hexalite 144
Hip, injuries to and around 85–92
  dislocations 88–90
  epiphyseal injuries 90–2
    complications 91
  fractures 85–7
  see also Femur
Humerus
  fractures 74, 76–7
    in children 132–3
  shaft 101

Hypovolaemic shock 125
Hypoxia 5

Injections causing injuries to vessels 108, 109
Injuries
  diagnosis, extent 6–7
  localised, diagnosing 6
  multiple, diagnosing 6–7
  see also Facial injuries; Head injuries
Intermittent Positive Pressure Respiration 22
Intraperitoneal bleeding, assessment 28
Intratracheal tube, inserting 5

Jugular vein, injuries 129–30

Kidney injuries 29
Knee injuries 93–4
  extensor 93
  fractures 94
  ligaments 93
  menisci 93
Kocher's manoeuvre 128

Lacerations
  conjunctiva 63
  ear 69
  effect on vessels 110
  eyelid 61–2
  limb 44
  throat and mouth 72
Lacrimal apparatus, injuries 68
Laparotomy 125–6
Larynx injuries 72
Le Fort I, II, and III fractures 12–13
  treatment 15–16
Leg injuries 44–6
  see also Limb, injuries
Ligaments, injuries 44–5
Limb
  injuries 44–6
    fractures 45
    lacerations 44, 45
    muscle 46
    peripheral nerves 46
    sprains 45
    vascular 45, 113–123
  ischaemia 111–12
  vascular injuries 113–23
    early management 113–15

Index

Limb — *cont.*
  vascular injuries — *cont.*
    operative management   115–22
    post-operative management   122–3
Liver injury   28
Long bones, fractures   101–3

Magnapen   49
Mandible, anatomy   12
  fractures   14–15
    treatment   16
March fracture   97
MAST   125
Metatarsal fractures   97
Middle third, facial skeleton, anatomy
    11–12
  fractures   12–13, 71
    treatment   15–16
Military Anti-Shock Trousers   125
Monitoring the patient's condition   54–7
  post-operative   122
Morphia administration   48–9, 52
  disadvantages   48–9
Mouth
  bleeding from, in head injuries   9
  injuries   72
  to mouth respiration   22
Muscle injury   46

Naloxone (Narcan) administration   49
Neck injuries   17–19
  cervical spine   17–19
  dislocation, management   19
  vascular   128–30
Neofract   144
Neurological injury, investigation   18
  skin and bladder care   18–19
Nitrous oxide/oxygen analgesia   47–8, 52
Nose
  bleeding in head injuries   9
  nose injuries   71
    foreign bodies   72
    fractures   71

Olecranon, fractures   78
Open fractures, treatment   136–7
Optic nerve injuries   68
Orbit, injuries   67–8
  fractures   67–8
  lacrimal apparatus   68
  nerve injuries   68
Orthotics   144–5

Os calcis, injuries   99–100
Osgood-Schlatter's disease   93
Otorrhoea   70
Outer ear   69

Palate, lacerations   72
Pancreas injury   30
Pelvic injury   32–41
  associated soft tissue typing   33–41
  closed injuries   39–40
  extraperitoneal rupture   40–1
  fractures   32–3
    classification   32
    treatment   32–3
  open injuries   39
Peripheral nerve injury   46
Peritonitis   30
  clinical signs   27
Phalanx, proximal, fracture in children
    134
Pharynx, injuries   72
Pinna, trauma, management   69
Pneumothorax   20, 21, 23
Post-operative management, abdominal
    injuries   122–3
  after amputation   143
Pringle's method   128
Prostacyclin in intra-arterial drug injection
    121
Pulse monitors   57
Pyelogram, intravenous   36

Radius fractures
  in children   134
  head   77
  shafts   101–2
Records, patients'   54
Renal failure following blood loss   111
Respiration, monitoring   56
Resuscitation   5
  in abdominal injuries   125
Ribs, fracture   20
  associated injuries   26
Rotator cuff, rupture   75

Scaphoid fracture   81
Scapula fracture   73
Septal haematoma   71
Shoulder, trauma to and around   73–5
  dislocation   74
Shunts, intraluminal   116–17

Index

Skull
  calipers 18
  injuries, investigations 9
Smith's fracture 80, 81
Soft tissue injuries
  ankle 95
  facial, treatment 16
  around wrist 79
Spasm, effect on vessels 109, 114
Spinal injuries
  cervical 17–19
  thoracolumbar 42
Spleen rupture 28–9
Splintage 144
Sprains 45
Staff, mobilisation 53
Steroid administration 51
Subclavian vessels, injuries 130
Sulphadimidine 49
Swan–Ganz catheter 58

Talus
  dislocation 98
    peritalar 98
  fractures 99
Tarsometatarsal joint dislocation 98
Temperature monitoring 58
Temporal bone fractures 69–70
Tendons, lacerated or ruptured 45
Tennis elbow 78
Tetanus, prophylaxis 50–1, 52
  toxoid 50, 51, 114
Thiopentone, intra-arterial injection 109, 113
  management 121–2
Thoracolumbar injuries 42–3
Thoracotomy
  emergency 125
  indications 23
Thorax in abdominal injuries 123–4, 125
Throat injuries 72
  foreign bodies 72
Thrombosis
  following accidental injection 113
  following blunt injury 109
Tibia and fibula, fractures 103
Tongue, lacerations 72
Trachea, ruptured 23
Tracheobronchial injuries 23
Tracheostomy, emergency 72
Traction effect on vessels 109
Transfusion, blood 31, 141

Trochanteric injuries 90–2
Tympanic membrane, rupture 69

Ulnar, shafts, fractures 101–2
Ureters, injury 31
Urethra
  female 38–9
  membranous 35–9
  rupture, male 33–5
    management 37–8
    with prostatic displacement 37
Urethrography 34, 36

Valium see Diazepam
Valoid see Cyclizine
Vascular injuries 107–31
  abdominal 123–8
  associated fractures 120–1
  associated injury 115
  effects 111–13
  fasciotomy 120
  limbs 113–23
  mechanisms 107–9
  neck 128–30
  types 107, 109–10
Vein
  graft 118–19
    failure 122–3
  injury, management 119
Vena cava repair 127
Ventilators 56
Vertebral arteries, injuries 129
Visceral damage 26–30
Volkmann's ischaemic contracture 112, 133

Wound care and debridement 117
Wrist, injuries to and around 79–82
  fractures 80–1
  non-penetrating injuries 80
  rehabilitation 81–2
  sprained 80

X-ray examination 7
  abdominal 27–8
  cervical spine 18–19
  diaphragm rupture 24
  elbow 76
  in vascular injury 115
  skull 9

Zygoma, fracture 14
  treatment 16